Making Love Better Than Ever

Praise for Dr. Barbara Keesling's work

"Finally here is a look at the overwhelmingly positive effects of sexual expression in our lives, including increased self-esteem, feelings of personal fulfillment and sexual ecstasy. Simplify your sex life and breathe some life back into that divinely sensual body."

— *Whole Life Times*

"In contrast to other how-to books about sex, which often focus on pleasing your partner at the expense of pleasing yourself, [Dr. Keesling] presents a series of meditative 'sensate focus' exercises designed to keep your attention on your own experience, without wandering off into anxious thoughts about what your partner might be experiencing. Solidly grounded in psychological, physiological, and experiential research, [Dr. Keesling] offers a reassuringly practical approach to enhancing the quality of sexual experiences."

— *Yoga Journal*

MAKING LOVE BETTER THAN EVER

Reaching New Heights *of* Passion *and* Pleasure After 40

Barbara Keesling, Ph.D.

Hunter House Inc., Publishers
An imprint of Turner Publishing Company
Nashville, Tennessee
www.turnerbookstore.com

Library of Congress Cataloging-in-Publication Data
Keesling, Barbara.
Making love better than ever : a guide to sexual pleasure / by Barbara Keesling. — 1st ed.
p. cm.
ISBN 9781630267865 (hardcover) — ISBN 9780897932318 (paperback)
1. Sex instruction. 2. Sex. 3. Love. 4. Man-woman relationships. I. Title.
HQ31.K385 1998'
613.9'6—dc21 98-20725
CIP

Development: Lisa E. Lee, Kiran Rana
Production: Wendy Low   Cover Design: Ame Beanland
Copyediting: Belinda Breyer   Editorial Assistance: Jennifer Huffaker
Proofreader: Susan Burckhard   Indexing: Kathy Talley-Jones
Marketing Director: Corrine M. Sahli   Special Sales Manager: Susan Markey
Customer Support: Christina Arciniega, Edgar M. Estavilla, Jr.
Order Fulfillment: A & A Quality Shipping
Publisher: Kiran S. Rana

Manufactured in the United States of America

9   8   7   6   5   4   3   2   First Edition

Contents

Acknowledgments

First of all, I would like to thank my clients. Much of what you have taught me is in this book, and I have learned more from you than you ever learned from me.

I would like to thank Michael Riskin, Anita Banker, Ron Gibb, James Gibbons, and all my former colleagues who developed a lot of the exercises in this book.

Special thanks to Lisa Lee, who was my editor at Hunter House for so long, and who still finds the best words for so many of the things I want to say.

Finally, I would like to thank everybody at Hunter House who worked on making and supporting this book, including Kiran Rana, Corrie Sahli, Wendy Low, Belinda Breyer, Susan Markey, Christina Arciniega, and Edgar Estavilla, Jr.

This book is dedicated to my clients

Important Note

Introduction

I n one or two earlier books I have written about my unusual background, and how it has given me the insights, qualifications, and inspiration to write books that foster healthy attitudes about sexuality. I grew up in a very restrictive religious family in Southern California. In 1980, while putting myself through college, I rebelled against these restrictions, decided to train as a surrogate partner, and began to work on a physical level with people who had sexual problems. Under the supervision of a sex therapist, I treated clients who had premature ejaculation and erection problems, as well as desire problems and problems sustaining relationships. I went on to earn a Ph.D. in Health Psychology at the University of California, and have taught college for many years since then.

The Evolution of Sexual Loving

In 1990 I published my first book, *Sexual Healing,* which focused on treating common but psychologically devastating sexual problems, including the inability to have orgasms, sexual anxiety, and ejaculation and erection problems. In that first book, I adapted typical exercises that surrogate partners do with their clients so that they could be used by couples at home. I eventually revised the book into a very different 1996 edition which focused on how intimate lovemaking can benefit a person's physical health and help heal emotional wounds. Along the way I wrote several other books, including *Sexual Pleasure: Reaching New Heights of Arousal and Intimacy* (the title says it all), *Talk Sexy to the One You Love* (about verbal cues for sexual arousal), *How to Make Love All Night* (about male multiple orgasm), and *Super Sexual Orgasm* (about female stimulation and arousal).

As I prepared to write this special book on the passions and pleasures of midlife loving, I said to myself, "Well, Barbara, you seem to have written about the full spectrum of male and female sexuality. What's missing?" And, of course, what has been missing is *love.* So I searched my extensive sexuality library to see who, if anyone, had dealt in depth with how your sexual relationship can deepen the love you have with your partner. I was surprised to find almost no books on this subject. The books on deepening love were nonsexual, and the books on sex (including my own, I must admit) really did not fully acknowledge this deep dimension of loving. I believe this omission is not because there is a lack of love in our relationships, but because most of us, especially when we are younger, find love is so difficult to define.

One of the college courses I teach is Social Psychology, which deals with how our thoughts, attitudes, and behavior are influenced by other people. Not surprisingly, two of the topics that social psychologists have studied in depth are attraction and love. *Making Love Better Than Ever* will introduce you to some of these psychological definitions of love, to help you better understand the nature of your relationship and what really brings the two of you together, connects you, both physically and emotionally. You will read this theoretical material about attraction, liking, and love in Chapter 1, in preparation for the specific loving exercises in the following twelve chapters.

Dimensions of Sexual Loving

With this book, I hope to reach and inspire people who want something *more* than just a sex manual—people who want to make love with their hearts, minds, and souls, not simply their bodies. Not surprisingly, writing this book has been more difficult than my other books, in part because of the intensely personal nature of the subject and in part because of the unique, intangible connection between love and sexuality.

In *Making Love Better Than Ever* I try to answer questions that are important to older, more mature couples, questions such as "How do I show the love I feel but find difficult to express sexually?" "How do I create more balance in the expression of sexual loving between us?" and "How can my partner of many years and I use lovemaking to find the spiritual dimension of our relationship?" While all my books are known for their practical advice, in this one I have tried to address the emotional layers of a relationship, specifically how to build a bridge between the expression of feelings and the intimate, sexual connection. I always offer down-to-earth exercises that really work—and you will find more of these here. I would even say that the secret door to sexual loving lies in these time-tested exercises, which have helped hundreds of my clients. But here more than ever I emphasize the *loving mindset,* the attitude toward each other and the commitment to doing this work together that can create a physical connection and an emotional intimacy between you that opens the way to profound sexual loving.

Who Can Use *Making Love Better Than Ever*

In general, *Making Love Better Than Ever* is for all adult couples who would like to deepen the love between them. The exercises have been very beneficial for couples who have a strong sexual bond and would like to use that bond to strengthen other aspects of their relationship. I am finding that they are also great for mature couples who have, for whatever reason, only now opened up to the idea of deepening their sexual engagement and passion. They provide a structure within which to develop gradual physical and emotional intimacy for those who are just beginning a new relationship.

Most of this book is written for couples. The foundation of any successful program of this kind, however, is an enhanced and properly understood self-love, which I see as self-respect combined with a full acknowledgment of our sexual and sensual dimension. For that reason, many of the exercises can be done by people currently without partners, just for themselves or in preparation for a relationship. And while I wrote *Making Love Better than Ever* with heterosexual couples in mind, the principles of the book and many of the exercises can be used by same-sex couples.

Embarking on the Loving Journey

Most of the chapters in this book involve exercises for you to do at home. Some have appeared in different forms in my previous books, many are new. As you approach them, try not to let the term "exercise" scare you away. To some the word suggests soulless techniques. Others are daunted by the prospect of some kind of sexual athletics. They aren't meant to be either, though it is really what you put into them together that will give them their character. You don't have to be especially physically fit to do any of these exercises, in fact the exercises themselves will increase your sexual fitness, pleasurably. They are not strenuous; they involve touch, sensuality, and sexuality. On the other hand, these exercises are not meant simply to improve sexual prowess. They are entryways to the great satisfaction that comes from a deeper appreciation of yourself, your lover, and your relationship.

To use the program in this book to best advantage, I ask you to give it a year. We have all realized by now that nothing worthwhile happens quickly or easily. It takes, so I'm told, about six months to learn to cook a decent omelet, eight years to become a doctor, and a lifetime to become a parent. A year is over before you know it—and think of the fun you will have! So do give it a year.

I suggest you both read the book completely through once, then go back to the beginning and start doing the exercises. Each chapter builds on earlier chapters, covering different aspects of your loving bond: touch and nonverbal communication, sexual pleasure and fulfillment, play and relaxation, and emotional intimacy.

Chapter 1, as I said, reviews psychological theories of love, attraction, and liking, and helps you develop the loving mindset. In Chapter 2, you will learn the importance of emotional bonding. Those of you embarking on new relationships can learn to create a loving bond and avoid previous relationship patterns right from the outset.

Chapters 3, 4 and 5 contain exercises you can do by yourself. They help you to convey love through your touch, and also teach you to convey that love to yourself.

Chapter 6 introduces techniques for sharing sensual and sexual exercises with your partner, while Chapter 7 shows you powerful, moving ways to experience intercourse.

Chapter 8 suggests ways to get back in touch with the joy and playfulness that enliven good lovemaking. In Chapter 9 you learn how to increase desire—an important topic for most couples in these days of rushed pleasures and dawn-to-dusk stress. And in Chapter 10 you will reintroduce loving words that have the power to shape, enhance, and convey your deepest desires during sessions of lovemaking.

Chapters 11 and 12 focus special attention on how to make love better than ever when one of you is dealing with a sexual problem or concern. Chapter 11 covers common concerns for men; Chapter 12 covers common concerns for women. Written for the partner of the person with the problem, these guides empower you to accept the challenge—and the privilege—of helping your partner with love and understanding. Finally, in Chapter 13, I bring you to the doorway of the sacred, the spiritual element of lovemaking, which can bring you and your partner in touch with something far greater than yourselves.

To derive the most benefit from *Making Love Better Than Ever*, I recommend that each partner do the self-exercises described in Chapters 3, 4, and 5. Some of these exercises (such as the PC muscle exercises) are done on a daily basis. You will probably feel like doing one or two other sensate focus exercises each week. There is no need to rush through this program. In fact, the slower you go, the more likely it is that the changes that occur in you as a result of this program will persist.

When you reach the stage (Chapters 6 and 7) where you are doing sensate focus exercises with your partner, you will probably feel like doing one or two exercises a week. Be sure to schedule time for each exercise so that you will not be interrupted. Feel free to go back any time and repeat an exercise if you liked it, or if you feel you were anxious and didn't get a lot out of it. Keep in mind that everyone and every couple advances at their own pace. Take the time to feel secure and comfortable with the beginning exercises before you jump into anything more advanced.

Also, make sure that you nourish your emotional and spiritual connection alongside your physical sexual abilities. If you skip the basics or try to take shortcuts in the advanced exercises, you will be shortchanging yourself—and your relationship. It takes care, focused attention, and gentle perseverance to nurture the loving powers of an intimate relationship.

Safe Sex

No book on sexuality is complete without a mention of safe sex. And safety, when it comes to sexuality, can mean a couple of things.

First, I have intended this book to be primarily for couples in a committed, monogamous, long-term relationship, because I believe that that kind of relationship is the setting in which the most powerful lovemaking can take place. So these exercises are written assuming a certain level of safety. However, I recognize that some of you may be in the beginning stages of a new relationship, or that you may not have a monogamous relationship.

While I prefer to focus on the positive aspects of making love, the reality of life today is that there are risks, no matter what your age. If you are in the beginning stages of a relationship, if you are not sure of your partner's past, of if you engage in high-risk behavior, please use condoms during any activities in which there is an exchange of body fluids. If you use condoms, make sure the lubrication you use is water-based, since oils will cause condoms to break. If your relationship and your commitment deepens, get tested for HIV antibodies and other sexually transmitted diseases to ensure that you both are free from sexual disease. Once those issues are accounted for you will feel closer, safer, and freer to make love without condoms.

Loving Communication

An important part of exploring these intimate, sexual exercises as a couple will be approaching them in a spirit of mutuality and trust. Respect each other's boundaries, give time to each other to deal with the habits and inhibitions of a lifetime. At the same time, be trusting and be adventurous. No one else is watching, so let go and try things you have always wanted to but might not have thought "proper." And talk! Spend time talking about each of the exercises in this book both before and after you have done them. As you work through the exercises in Chapters 2 through 12, take a few minutes after each exercise to relax together and talk about it. Be open in your discussion, and try to avoid your usual ways of communicating. Focus on each other as you talk, respect each other's energy levels and emotions. Listen intently and don't interrupt. Ask each other questions along these lines: How did you feel during the exercise? Which part of the exercise was most enjoyable for you? What percent of the time were you able to concentrate during the touching? Is there anything about the exercise you didn't like? Would you like to do this exercise again? What changes would you like to make?

In time, the enhanced communication with your partner will become another profound and deeply rewarding benefit of the year—or lifetime—you spend making love better than ever.

Chapter 1

Making Love Better Than Ever

Having sex is a purely physical act. Making love involves all aspects of our person and who we are. Making love brings together our bodies, our minds, our emotions, and our spirits and seeks to join them in union with our partner. Our passion is the psychological state of arousal that makes this union happen.

The main idea behind *Making Love Better Than Ever* is twofold: Loving your partner makes your sexual relationship better, and having great passionate sex will cause you to fall in love with your partner all over again.

9

Making Love Better Than Ever is full of fun, sensual, loving exercises that you and your partner can do together to create what I call "sexual loving." But before introducing any of these exercises, I would like to discuss the difference between falling in love and staying in love, and what it takes to create the kind of loving *sexual* bond that can sustain a relationship over many years.

In this chapter we will look at the most influential psychological theories of attraction, liking, and loving. This is not meant to be a critique or a display of scholarship. I want to get you thinking about which factors have been important or relevant in *your* relationship. Think back about the time when you first met your partner: What drew you together? How and why did you fall in love? Why did you decide to make the relationship permanent—or did you?

As you read this chapter, ask yourself: Are those same qualities present now? Are they what you cherish about each other? What factors would you like to see in your relationship that are not there now?

If you have a solid relationship, this book will help you to deepen your passion and open the door to greater sexual wisdom. If you started your relationship on the wrong foot or if you feel your relationship has deteriorated, it's not too late! You can learn to re-create and express deep love through the exercises described in these pages and the trust, commitment, and passion they engender.

Theories about Love

There is a lot of confusion about love (as well there should be, as no one knows what it really is!). And there are almost as many theories about love as there are people who have fallen in love. Psychologists, poets, philosophers, moviemakers, even biochemists have tried to get to the bottom of this unique, transcendent, and often agonizing human experience. To help you get some insights into the quality and longevity of your relationship, let's look at the theories of attraction, liking, and loving that are rooted in psychology. Then we can take the best parts of these theories and see how they relate to you.

Factors in Attraction

There are a number of factors that have been reliably shown to foster our attraction to another person. Some of these factors are quite shallow, and are based on short-term perceptions or needs. Unfortunately, many people use these factors to determine whether they should start a relationship or make love with a potential mate. Each of these factors acts as a sort of filter or stage—you don't reach the next one until you've passed through the previous one.

Proximity

Many people overlook this obvious fact, but the first factor in initial attraction is *proximity*. There is a high degree of correlation between being in the presence of a person and being attracted to that person. The more often you are near someone, the more likely it is that an attraction will grow.

Familiarity

We tend to be more attracted to people and things that we are exposed to frequently. This is sometimes called the "mere exposure" effect. Whether it is a song on the radio, a television show, or a person, the more familiar something is, the more easily we are attracted to it.

Physical Attractiveness

Most of us are attracted to people who are good-looking, and most of us can successfully judge the degree of another person's physical attractiveness within our culture. In today's American culture, for example, this means that men, in general, are attracted to women with even facial features, good hair, good teeth, and a certain waist-to-hip ratio. Women, in general, are attracted to men who are taller than average and have broad shoulders and strong facial features. Individual people have individual preferences, but these general preferences have been bred into us over thousands of years. In addition, we tend to be attracted to people we perceive as being similar to ourselves in appearance.

Need for Affiliation

We also tend to be attracted to other people when we have a psychological need to be with or around someone else. This need to affiliate can be caused by fear, insecurity, or both. If we are in a psychological state of needing or wanting affiliation—perhaps due to some extreme event that has deprived us of human companionship—we may find people attractive that we would not find attractive under normal circumstances.

Factors in Liking

Attraction is a psychological process, and doesn't require verbal contact. We often become attracted to people we have seen but have had no further contact with. When we do have further contact, factors involved in *liking* come into play.

Social psychologists believe that most of us process fairly complex information about other people quite quickly to decide whether we like them or not.

Some of the hundreds of different qualities we notice when we come into contact with another person are: physical attractiveness, body language, intelligence, or specific status symbols worn or used by that person. We notice a person's state of physical and mental health. We may actually even subliminally register—quite strongly—how a person smells. We are also aware of whether a person is responding positively to us or not.

Other information we take into account includes such things as a person's personality traits, their apparent emotional make-up, the nature of their self-disclosure, and their perceived similarities to ourselves. Some of the key factors are discussed further below.

Cultural Factors

Cultural factors influence our initial perceptions as well. For example, research shows that within ten seconds of meeting a person for the first time we have made judgments about that person's social status based on clothing, jewelry, or automobile, depending on what status symbols are valued in our cultural context. For example, in a certain social milieu, wearing Birkenstock sandals and not shaving your legs (if you are a woman) may actually be a status symbol, and help you to fit in. In a chic resort town the opposite would probably be the case.

The main thing to remember about cultural factors is that they are very important in our relationships and in our deciding whether we are in love and want to have sex, but they are the factors that we are *most* likely to ignore or not be aware of. Like the fish that doesn't know it is wet, we are so immersed in our culture that we are unaware of how profoundly it influences our perceptions and our relationships. (This is what's called a "nonconscious ideology.")

The best way to understand how your culture influences your relationship is to study relationships in other cultures and realize that if you lived in another country or historical period, your assumptions about relationships would be completely different. Those of you who have relationships that cross cultural, ethnic, and geographical boundaries have probably experienced this already.

Body Language

Body language, or nonverbal communication, is the medium through which most of us get information about another person's emotional make-up. Whether consciously or not, we notice things like facial expressions, tone of voice, gestures, and posture to determine whether we like a person or not. Some people have intense personal *charisma*—nonverbal qualities that draw others to them. Still others fake nonverbal expressiveness in order to hide their true feelings, or to make a calculated impression on others. Part of our body language readings includes whether we feel someone's nonverbal responses are genuine or not.

Self-Disclosure

Self-disclosure refers to the process by which we verbally share information about ourselves with another. There are four basic levels of self-disclosure, each level becoming progressively more intimate. When two people first meet they tend to share information about personal taste, such as taste in art or music. Once they become more comfortable and familiar with each other, they share information or personal opinions on weightier or more controversial subjects, such as politics and religion. The third level of intimacy involves discussing one's self-concept, how one sees oneself. The highest level of self-disclosure, not surprisingly, involves sharing sexual information about ourselves.

In general, people like other people who are high self-disclosers, unless they disclose highly personal or "weird" information too early in a relationship. We also tend to like people who disclose at the same level at which we ourselves are comfortable disclosing.

At that sensitive point in a relationship when we begin to self-disclose, we usually become more acutely aware of similarities and differences between the other person and ourselves. On some level, we begin to consider our compatibility, the philosophical value of our relationship, and the potential for a deepening, intimate relationship.

Similarity

Similarity is perhaps the strongest factor in liking. It is the factor that holds together many friendships, and is usually the best predictor of longevity in romantic relationships. We tend to like people who look like us, share similar tastes, and have similar backgrounds such as age, religion, or ethnicity. The most important similarities that contribute to relationship satisfaction and longevity are similarities in personality, attitudes, core values, and role definitions. These points are the crux of what makes or breaks love relationships. Not surprisingly, we choose our friends according to whether they are similar to us in these areas, too.

For some people, particularly at adolescence and other times of marked growth or reexamination, the initial point of attraction to a partner is that they are an opposite, or "other." Sometimes we are attracted to people who are different from us because of the novelty. For example, a shy or introverted person may be attracted to a potential partner who is perceived to be outgoing and gregarious. Or a straight-laced person may have an initial attraction to a partner who appears uninhibited and impulsive.

Notice I said that this is a factor in *initial* attraction. Whether this attraction of opposites, which is called "complementarity," predicts a positive future for the relationship depends on whether these initial appearance and body language factors are a reflection of deeper personality traits or whether they are a relatively shallow reflection of social trends.

I think that sooner or later people who are usually attracted to opposites analyze their relationship failures and realize that they would be better off with someone similar to themselves. I also think the reasons some of us are attracted to opposites are boredom and perceived inadequacy or dissatisfaction with some aspect of our appearance or personality.

So—if you like someone who is like you, your chances of having a long-term relationship are better. Opposites attract, but similarity has staying power.

| Similarity → | Liking → | Long term |
| Opposites → | Initial attraction → | Fades out |

Of course there are situations in which similarity does not predict longevity, for example if you have huge amounts of external stress on the relationship. For people over forty this kind of stress often comes from different ideas on dealing with growing children, differences about sharing money, and issues of personal betrayal. In that case even similarity and liking may not be able to hold the relationship together.

Reinforcement

"Reinforcement" is the idea that we like another person based on the rewards that being with that person brings us. These rewards are usually not material but social—laughter and good times, positive feedback, enhanced creativity, and so forth. According to Reinforcement Theory, the more rewards a relationship provides, the more we will like the person involved. Conversely, the more negative outcomes that occur in conjunction with a person, the less we will like that person.

Reinforcement Theory predicts that if I feel okay and an attractive partner comes along, I will feel better. If I feel lonely and an attractive partner comes along, I will feel *even* better, because that person has not only made me feel good but has also removed the source of my pain.

One aspect of this is that falling in love may have as much to do with your mental state as it does with any of the characteristics of your partner. Reinforcement can also be unhealthy if we see our partner only as the source of relief of our misery and not as an individual. In that case we will become dependent.

Social Exchange

Exchange Theory grows out of the idea that we all have certain assets that we exchange with another person in a relationship. These assets might be money, physical attractiveness, social power, information, nurturing, affection, caring, or just about anything. According to the theory of social exchange, then, the more ways we benefit from being around a person, either by increased affection or social status, the greater our attraction to that person.

For some couples, this is why their differences can make them stronger. One partner may provide what the other lacks and vice versa. Over time each person develops a liking or a tolerance for those opposite traits in their partner. For other couples, a relationship based on social exchange can become limiting or burdensome, and resentment can develop toward the partner and the relationship.

Physiological Theories of Love

You may be excited to hear that love at first sight isn't a myth. While we may not be able to explain such experiences, which sometimes run counter to intellect and common sense, we've all had them. There are a number of theories that attempt to explain the intense physiological arousal and psychological absorption that occur in the "hit-by-a-lightning-bolt" experience.

What the physiological theories of love all have in common is their most basic assumption that the root of love is some kind of change in the body, for example, a hormone change that causes our heart to race or our brain to release endorphins (pleasure chemicals). In these theories love is primarily a physical experience.

Misattribution

According to the Misattribution Theory of love, all our emotions consist of two components: physical arousal and a cognitive label. For example, let's say you are crossing the street and all of a sudden a truck you didn't notice before comes barreling around the corner, threatening to run you over. Your adrenaline starts to flow, your heart pounds, and you breathe rapidly. This is physical arousal. What you feel—the label that you give your experience—is the emotion "fear."

The main idea behind the Misattribution Theory of love is that if we meet a potential love partner when we are highly aroused and aren't sure why, we may attribute our arousal to the presence of that person, making them a potential love object. Taking the truck example again, let's say someone saved you from the truck just as it was about to run you over. The danger would have caused a high state of arousal, which might spill over in how you respond to your rescuer, who you then might see as courageous and attractive and promptly "fall in love" with.

Lest you think that misattribution only occurs in extreme situations, consider the circumstances under which most couples today are likely to meet. These situations—a health club, a nightclub, a party or social event, an exciting movie—involve high levels of physical arousal and may also involve the release of endorphins through physical exertion or the use of alcohol or other drugs. It is very possible that many of us fell in love with our current partners to some degree because we initially spent time with them in physically arousing but nonsexual situations.

Biochemical Theories

Biochemists believe that the feeling of being in love has to do with the presence of certain chemicals in our bodies called *pheromones*. Pheromones are similar to hormones but they are secreted outside the body. The mating of most animals involves the intricate release of and response to pheromones. Recent research also shows that humans perceive pheromones without being conscious of it and are attracted to members of the opposite sex if they subliminally like their smell. (Could there be such as thing as love at first smell?) This seems to be especially true for women, who appear to be "turned off" or unconsciously repulsed by the smell of certain males. In fact, research has discovered that women have a larger number of pheromone receptors in their nasal tissues than men. How's that for evolutionary difference?

Evolutionary Theory

Evolutionary theories of attraction and love are currently quite popular with psychologists. The main idea is that we are attracted to members of the opposite sex who we perceive as healthy because they could become fit mothers or fathers for our offspring. This theory holds that love then develops as a way to keep a procreative couple together and to guarantee that their offspring would be protected and live to reproductive age.

Psychological Theories of Love

What the psychological theories of love have in common is the basic assumption that love is primarily psychological or mental and that physiological states are not so important. There is a suggestion that you can rationally analyze love, and that if certain conditions occur or certain factors add up, you will decide that you are in love.

Liking and Loving

This theory, proposed by social psychologist Zick Rubin, holds that "liking" and "loving" are two separate dimensions of feeling between partners that can occur together or independently. In other words, you could potentially love your partner without particularly liking him or her. According to Rubin, *love* has three components—intimacy, possessiveness, and preoccupation—whereas *liking* consists of similarity and respect. The main nonverbal differences that Rubin found between couples who say they like each other and couples who say they are in love is that the couples who are "in love" touch each other and gaze into each other's eyes more.

Triangular Theory

In psychologist Robert Sternberg's Triangular Theory, the three components of love are *intimacy, passion,* and *commitment.* Consummate love, or fully realized love, has all three components—intimacy, which is emotional and verbal closeness; passion, which is erotic love or lust; and behavioral commitment. However, it is very possible that a relationship might only have two of these three components. For example, if a couple have passion and intimacy but no commitment, they have "romantic" love. If a couple have passion and commitment but no intimacy, they have "fatuous" (or foolish) love. If a couple have intimacy and commitment but no passion, they have "companionate" love.

A relationship might also have only one of the components. If a couple just have intimacy, their connection might be considered a liking relationship, similar to a friendship. If they have only passion, they have infatuation. And if they only have commitment, as in many arranged marriages, they have what Sternberg would call "empty" love.

This Triangular Theory of love seems to be one of the best thought-out theories on this complex subject. According to my experience and the research of others it also has value in predicting whether couples will stay together. Couples who share the richness and balance of all three types of love create the kind of union that lasts through the years. Other couples who have only one or two aspects of love may work to round out their relationships, or they may feel dissatisfied on some level, and eventually break up.

Lovestyles

The "lovestyles" approach to relationships was developed by sociologist J.A. Lee, and expanded by two psychologists, Hendrick and Hendrick. The idea behind lovestyles is that love means different things to different people, and there are different types of love. Lee uses Greek words to define the different lovestyles, the primary ones being *eros* (erotic, passionate love), *ludus* (game-playing love), and *storge* (friendship love). Secondary lovestyles are *pragma* (practical, shopping-list love), *mania* (possessive or obsessive love), and *agape* (altruistic or selfless love).

When partners define love in different ways, problems arise in relationships. One of the clearest examples of mismatching lovestyles is when one partner defines love as physical, passionate love and the other partner defines love in practical terms. "Do you love me?" she asks. He answers, "Well, I mowed the lawn today, didn't I?" (This is the "Venus and Mars" issue.) Given their lovestyles, this couple is instinctively primed for misinterpreting each other's comments and behavior as unaffectionate, demanding, and sarcastic. Conscious knowledge, acceptance of the other's style of love, and the willingness to keep "translating" will help them avoid conflicts.

Psychoanalytic Theories

Psychoanalytic theory was first developed by Sigmund Freud, who proposed the idea that unconscious conflicts power our behavior and are very powerful in the area of love and intimate relationships. Psychoanalytic theories of love hold that we fall in love based on unconscious needs that originate in our childhood relationships with our parents. This is called Attachment Theory—the idea that in order to love completely as an adult we must form an emotional bond with a caregiver when we are infants. If we do so successfully, we form what is called a secure attachment and are capable of complete love as an adult.

If our primary bond with our caregiver was unhealthy in some way, this will play itself out in all our loving relationships. For example, if our caregiver neglected us we may become avoidant in future relationships, and if our caregiver was alternately abusive and overprotective, we may find that we are anxious or ambivalent in future relationships.

Cultural and Social Theories

Unique factors in our culture and society, not surprisingly, affect our love relationships and our sex lives. In a society in which men outnumber women, women are likely to be valued and the societal ethos is likely to favor romance. But in societies in which women outnumber men, sex or procreation is valued over romance and men see women as status symbols, as property, or as low-level labor.

There are a number of sources for cultural and social beliefs. Communications and the mass media create and sustain some of them. Social institutions, such as organized religion, the military, government, and business create others. Others evolve from art, literature, and philosophy—in fact, some cultural and social beliefs can be traced to specific works of literature and philosophy. Most cultural and social beliefs, however, are complex and have evolved over time.

Certain aspects in our Western culture favor the development of certain schemas or mental frameworks for love, romance, and sex. For example, in American society television and movies are quite influential in generating stereotypes of love situations. A common stereotype is the "star-crossed lovers". (Lest you think this idea went out in Shakespeare's day, as I write this the film *Titanic* has been the top-grossing movie for several weeks in a row and holds the Academy Award record for 14 Oscars!)

Romantic love as the basis for having sex or for getting married is not the norm in every culture. We equate sex and love in this culture, but many cultures don't. Even in this culture, the idea that you should be "in love" with someone before you get married and have sex is a fairly recent, twentieth-century development. Prior to that marriages were based on a potential spouse's "suitability" for marriage—on practical factors such as social status, property, and social necessity. Many cultures around the globe still have arranged marriages. You may find it very interesting to know that when these arranged marriages are based on similarity of background and similar attitudes toward roles in relationships, they tend to be very successful.

The Conventional Wisdom

When couples who have been together happily for many years are asked, "What is the secret of the longevity of your relationship?" the two factors they mention most often are initial physical attraction and a mutual respect that has developed over the years. When asked to define "respect," these couples usually explain that it involves not only treating your partner the way you would want to be treated, but treating your partner the way you treat yourself.

Insights

Now that you are familiar with the different theories of love, let's draw some conclusions that will be important in helping you develop the *sexual loving mindset* that will help you learn to make love better than ever. Hopefully, this review has you thinking about which factors have been important or relevant in *your* relationship. Think back about the time when you first met your partner and why you chose a permanent relationship with him or her. Are those same qualities present now? What factors would you like to see in your relationship that are not present now? How and why did you fall in love with your partner?

Even if you started your relationship on the wrong foot, or even if your relationship has deteriorated to the point where it has only one of Sternberg's components, it's not too late! The ideas and exercises in this book can still help you learn to deepen your bond with your partner and express greater love through lovemaking.

One of the first things I notice about all of these theories is that none of them mention sex! The Triangular and Lovestyles theories both mention "passion," which we can take to be their euphemism for sex. But this lack of a coherent approach to sex in any of these theories reflects the fact that scientists are reluctant to study sex in any context other than sexual behavior. As I write, the media are full of survey findings that indicate that highly-educated people tend to have less sex than people who are not as well-educated. I find statistics like this to be meaningless. They tell us nothing about what is really important: Are certain groups of people enjoying their lovemaking more? Does lovemaking means different things to different groups of people? Are certain groups of people pleased and satisfied with their lovemaking?

I am not aware of any research that attempts to study and make conclusions about this relationship between love and sex, or which components of loving and liking lead to better sex and vice versa. And since there is no current theory that brings this together, I'd like to share with you my own.

Mutuality, Intimacy, Commitment, and Passion

Sharing similar attitudes and values seems to be essential for the success of a "liking" relationship. For lovers, however, while liking can sustain a relationship, it can't be everything. *Mutuality, intimacy, commitment* and *passion* are the cornerstones of a profound and perpetual love. They are the foundation that you will set down as you begin making love better than ever.

The exercises in this book will teach you ways to access and develop these four qualities in your relationship. You will learn to promote mutuality (movement toward common goals) because in the exercises you spend extended periods of time paying attention to the same thing at the same time, both totally focused on the here and now. The physical closeness and shared trust you experience during the exercises will lead to emotional closeness, which will deepen your intimacy. As you pay attention to and spend time with each other's bodies, and learn to talk intimately about sexual matters, you will become closer than ever to each other.

There are two ways in which the exercises contribute to strengthening your commitment. The first is that a big part of making a commitment to each other is committing to *change*. We get older, we grow wiser, and we evolve from our experiences—we are dynamic processes, and our relationships must change as we do. You have picked up this book because you want the richness of sexual loving in your relationship. To create that you must acknowledge and celebrate the dynamic evolution of your selves and each other. And *that* is a commitment to change.

The second way in which the exercises help to develop commitment is that when you agree to do an exercise together at a certain time, and you actually follow through and do the exercise you have agreed on, you are learning commitment in small, painless steps. A lifetime of keeping your commitments is what earns you the respect of your partner.

So what about passion, the potentially most powerful component of your love relationship? Even if there hasn't been passion in your relationship for some time, you can get it back. Passion leads to great lovemaking, *but great lovemaking also creates passion.* Whatever you do, don't wait until you feel passion to do the powerful exercises on arousal and orgasm that follow in this book. Create your passion by reaching these heights of arousal and orgasm together. Your physical sexual union is the best way you have to create, express, and communicate love.

The Loving Mindset

I don't believe that there is any place in a love relationship for jealousy, possessiveness, game playing, manipulation, or obsession. Our marriages and romantic partnerships should be a place where we can be truly selfless, offering up our love and nurturing to another. They should be a haven where we find self-expression, enjoy the unbridled encouragement of another, and discover new aspects of our self. Our loving relationships should be partnerships, filled with rich, resonant love.

Most exercises in Making Love Better Than Ever involve a great deal of touch. Through them, I hope you will come to a new understanding of the power that touch has to convey and kindle our emotions—and our connection with another. As you do these exercises, focus specifically on your touch. Pour into it your full *attention*, and your full *intention*.

As you stroke and caress each other, keep the following qualities in the forefront of your mind. These are the qualities that you want your touch to convey:

- Mutuality
- Intimacy
- Commitment
- Passion
- Acceptance
- Lust
- Selflessness

Review this list before you do any exercise. If it seems awkward or complicated to you at first, try to convey one quality at a time. When you are able to convey all of these things to your partner (and to yourself) through your touch, you will truly know what it means to *make love better than ever!*

Chapter 2
Building the Foundation of a Loving Relationship

A re you beginning a new relationship? Or are you reading this book with the intention of renewing the passion and energy of your marriage? Perhaps you have simply entered a new phase brought on by the changes that hit us in mid-life—children leaving home, retirement, physical and hormonal changes—and are taking the opportunity to reinvent your relationship.

All of these situations offer you and your partner the opportunity to develop the intimacy, mutuality, commitment, and love that will lay the groundwork for a loving relationship that will grow old with you. For those of you who are married, the exercises in this chapter will help you get to know each other anew and to fall in love again. And for those of you who are just starting out in a relationship, your first step is to make sure you have chosen the right partner, then to create loving ways of relating.

Is There Really a Mr. Right?

Inevitably, as you embark on a new relationship you will consider whether the relationship has the capacity for a lifetime of love. We have all heard the expression, "Once bitten, twice shy." It's wise to be cautious, but don't let past experiences breed cynicism or insecurity. Instead, draw on them to educate your common sense and reaffirm your gut instincts.

How do you distinguish a potential loving and intimate life partner from one who will bail at the first sign of trouble? How do you know who is for real and who is not?

There are definite warning signs for the *wrong* person: verbal or emotional abuse, dishonesty, criticism, addiction, and especially physical violence. But there are other, less obvious signs that you might overlook in the throes of newness or attraction. Does this relationship make you anxious or depressed? Does your partner manipulate you? Does he or she cling with dependency, or withdraw during disagreement without discussion or compromise? Do you feel an imbalance of power in the relationship? If you have not made a commitment to this relationship, and these issues have appeared, it is best to get out now.

Many of the warning signs become obvious once you have a certain amount of experience with relationships—your own and others. But what do you look for beyond this? Most people start relationships for the wrong reasons, based on the principles of attraction discussed in the last chapter: emotional needs, vulnerability, physical attraction, social status, and so forth. Unfortunately, none of these qualities really predicts whether a couple will share a growing, evolving love. This may sound old-fashioned, but when considering a true partner you have to look for qualities of character and values above all else. These are the ones that time and again lead to satisfaction in love and a relationship that lasts.

It can be difficult to judge another person's character, especially if you don't give yourself time and don't see the person in the different situations of his or her normal life. Even though our instincts are often correct, we may have developed a habit of not paying attention to them. Or we may feel pressured—by loneliness, advancing age, family or peer pressure, or the difficulty of just meeting people—to find someone. As I suggested in the last chapter, one of the keys is to find people who are like you, who do and enjoy the same things, who share the same interests and values. This suggests looking for a partner in your "natural habitat"—the places you usually go, doing the things you usually do.

The next thing is to try to assess the values of your potential partner. If I wanted to start a relationship with a person, I would want to know not *what* that person had achieved but *why*. If your lifelong goals are intimacy, mutuality, commitment, and love, who is a better relationship bet, someone who refers to his ex-wife as a shrew or someone who makes an effort to get along with a difficult ex-spouse so that his kids have a stable life? Someone who works to help her children get through school and get good grades, or someone who spends evenings drinking and partying because someone else is paying for it? Habits of character are ingrained early. Can you imagine a world in which the people with good character were the most valued and sought after for relationships rather than the best-looking people?

Boy Meets Girl, Boy Gets Girl, Then What?

Let's look at a couple of typical case histories, using the theories of love and attraction we talked about in Chapter 1. Some of us are able to navigate the treacherous waters of romance and find a decent part-ner. But a lot of us are looking for partners using the wrong criteria (looks, money, status, and so forth), and many others are facing life partners chosen at too early an age.

Consider the dynamics that typically occur with young couples. The following scenario is taken from one of my previous books, *Sexual Healing,* and typifies the couples I see in therapy.

Melissa and *David* begin dating in their late teens. Aside from a few dalliances, neither is very sexually experienced. Both live with their parents. They date for all the "right" reasons: they are similar in looks and personality, and appear to have a lot in common. At some point David pressures Melissa into having sex, and they have it when they can—often in his car. There isn't much foreplay, and sex is over quickly. Melissa doesn't really enjoy the sex, although it gets some-what better as the relationship progresses, but she feels that they have become closer.

When the two reach a certain age and have been together for a number of years, they experience a lot of social pressure to marry. So they do. After twenty years of marriage they find themselves with two teenage children and stressed out. Work, school, and the kids have taken priority over the time they once spent together. They have little time for lovemaking, and are often too tired anyway. Out of boredom, isolation, or alienation, one or both have an affair, and they think sex with their new lover is the greatest they have ever had. When they divorce, everyone says, "What a shame. They must have grown apart."

The truth is that they were never really together. Melissa and David's relationship reached a peak of intimacy when they were still dating, just about the time before they first had sex. That was when they felt closest to each other. They may have reached another peak of intimacy when they had their first child. But as they went about their day-to-day lives, they missed communicating and sharing with each other, growing together, and making love. As a result their rela-tionship became less and less intimate over time.

David and Melissa's story is fairly typical, and it is worth asking what went wrong in their relationship. When they started dating, neither David nor Melissa knew very much, if anything, about his or her own body or how to relate sexually and intimately to a lover. It is not a matter of whether they had sex too early in the relationship or whether they were too young when they first had sex (only they can say). The problem was that they never let real intimacy develop— slowly and solidly—between them.

We can analyze David and Melissa's relationship in terms of the theories of love and attraction in Chapter 1. They probably never went past the surface attraction factors like looks and similarity in tastes. Only one of them (David) had passion in the relationship to begin with. In terms of Sternberg's Triangular Theory of love, they began their relationship with fatuous love and ended up with empty love—a commitment only. In terms of the theory behind this book, they had no intimate, loving sexual bond to provide novelty, warmth, and mutuality in their relationship. No wonder they got divorced.

Let us look at another typical scenario. *Paula* and *Jerry* meet through work (proximity and familiarity). They are attracted to each other's looks. Both of them have just broken up from previous relationships and are eager to start another relationship. In terms of theories of attraction they both have a high need for affiliation. But the most important factor in their initial attraction is a perceived similarity in background, attitudes, personality, and values, and they develop a strong liking for each other.

Paula and Jerry are both in their early forties and are self-confident lovers who enjoy passionate and frequent sex. Because they are older and more experienced they have sex on their first date and move in together within a month. Again, their relationship progresses according to outward signs; they marry shortly and have a child. Although everything else in the relationship is good, the sex soon becomes pretty lousy, not to mention infrequent. Eventually they both experience a lack of desire; they feel bored and unsatisfied, they miss the passion they once felt. These feelings begin to permeate other aspects of their relationship, and pretty soon Paula and Jerry divorce.

What happened here? This couple started with high levels of both liking and passion or erotic love. Life changes caused their sex drives to decrease, and somehow they did not have the intimate, loving, sexual bond to connect their liking and passion and sustain the relationship. They had both been running purely on hormones and were unprepared for what happened when those hormones were no longer driving their sexual behavior.

How about a third couple with a slightly different outcome? *Janie* and *Bob* met at a singles dance when they were in their late forties. They had both been divorced from other partners and had children in college. They had a strong perceived similarity and liked each other a great deal. Both of their first marriages had been quite sexual, and they both unconsciously harbored a belief that "great sex equals a lousy marriage in other ways." Bob and Janie made love, moved in together, and eventually married after five years of very comfortable cohabiting.

Neither of them felt a particularly strong erotic or passionate sexual bond. In their fifties, when their sexual desire decreased, they just stopped having sex. They did not have the experience of an intense, intimate, erotic sexual bond to sustain them during the hormonal dry periods that every couple inevitably faces. However, still in love with each other and satisfied with the life they had built together, they settled for a life of companionate love, which is what a lot of people do.

Why do I sound as if I've heard these stories a million times? Because I have. These are *the* typical experiences that people relate when, instead of divorcing, they come in for sex therapy. I teach them how to cultivate that loving, intimate, passionate bond and how to make love better than ever so that their sexual loving can sustain their relationship.

In all of these scenarios the couple reached a peak level of sexual activity much too early in the relationship and lost it steadily thereafter. They expected that the sexual charge they achieved when first dating (when the hormones were really flowing) would and should be the norm for sex throughout their lives. It won't be. It can't be. People grow and change, and so does their sexual expression.

The good news is that this growth can bring you and your lover closer together. Your relationship *can* improve, and you *can* experience deeper and richer passion as you grow older together—if you work toward it by building intimacy, mutuality, commitment, and love.

What Happens When We Begin Again?

It's difficult enough starting a new relationship when we are young and relatively inexperienced. But sometimes that shared inexperience allows you to grow together and brings you closer. It's even more difficult to begin a new relationship after being intimate with only one person for a number of years, especially when you consider that second and third marriages statistically stand less of a chance of longevity than first marriages.

What issues are common and unique to men and women who begin new relationships after being with one person for a long time? In addition to being open to things like physical attractiveness and similarity, you may both be carrying a lot of baggage from your first relationship. Some of the factors people contemplating second relationships have to deal with include whether or not they have children, whether they have strong family and community ties, the amount of sexual experience they had prior to their first monogamous relationship, their body image, their degree of self-knowledge, whether their first relationship was negative or abusive, who ended the prior relationship, and whether they are seeking to correct a specific deficiency from the previous relationship. People who have neglected their physical appearance or become complacent in their previous relationship may also experience intense performance anxiety at the thought of starting a new relationship.

Recent research shows that the people who adjust best to beginning a new relationship later in life are those who look toward the future and see the potential and possibilities rather than those who constantly compare the new relationship with the previous one. In addition, people who were capable of a sustained intimate, erotic, sexual relationship in the past seem more likely to be successful in a second relationship.

Taking the Time You Need to Get It Right

The most important thing you can do when embarking on a new relationship, one that you hope will include love, is to make sure you get intimate with the right person for the right reasons. Be honest and true to yourself above all else. Is this someone you like and respect? Are you friends? Are you looking to fill a need, or are you ready for love? Do you accept your pasts and are you ready to build your future—together? If so, then progress in your conversation and physical involvement to increasingly more intimate areas.

Keep in mind that both verbal self-disclosure and physical intimacy occur at several levels. When people first meet socially they talk about their tastes—their likes and dislikes—such as in movies or music. Unfortunately, most people halt the level of intimate conversation right there. But as you know, loving relationships that last through the years are based on deeper sharing, caring, and understanding. A deeper level of verbal intimacy is reached when opinions and feelings are shared on value-driven areas such as politics and religion. An even more intimate level is reached when we share emotionally charged material about how we see ourselves, what we think of ourselves. The highest level of verbal intimacy includes sharing feelings about sex, possibly including guilt, shame, or inadequacies.

If you have been through relationships once, twice, or a few times before, you may find it easy to hop into a relationship with a potential partner. On the other hand, you may feel out of touch with the dating scene, and pursue what seems easiest or the least uncomfortable. Older women, in particular, may fall prey to the "settle for" syndrome, while older men often try to recreate a relationship more appropriate to their younger days.

If you are just starting out in a relationship and you want emotional closeness to grow throughout your relationship, take time to develop intimacy through verbal disclosure. Also make sure there is always some aspect of physical lovemaking that you have yet to try. Physical intimacy also progresses in stages. I tend to think of these stages as: no physical contact; sharing something physical together, such as a sport; the nonsexual touching that goes on between friends, such as a hug or a kiss on the cheek; sexual touch; intercourse; and orgasm. It is truly rare and wonderful when you can share all levels of verbal intimacy and physical intimacy with one person. But some people try to do it all in one night! That seldom—or never—works, it really isn't fun or meaningful, and it's a lousy foundation for a lasting relationship.

If you and your partner take the time and make the space necessary for emotional intimacy, you will find that vistas of unexplored sexual expression will unfold for you. Similarly, if you constantly look for new perspectives and new areas of self-disclosure you will always have something to talk about. Don't you think it's a shame when you see an older couple in public and they are clearly having the same exact discussion or argument they have been having for fifty years, with the same result? Do you feel worse when you realize that it could be you?

Exercises for Opening to Intimacy

The exercises in this chapter create and strengthen emotional bonds between lovers. In the social sciences, "bonding" usually refers to the emotional connection that develops between a child and a caregiving parent. A vital, intimate bond is created by parents through spending a lot of time cuddling and holding, nurturing and playing with their child. These activities give a child the love, security, and self-worth necessary to venture out into the world and mature fully.

As adults we can bond with each other too. The following exercises create and strengthen those intimate, bonding feelings. But be forewarned—don't try these with your partner unless you really do want to become closer. They will help you become relaxed with each other, and attuned to your heart rhythms. They will help express how you accept your partner and help you feel accepted. It is easy to tell your partner, "I love you," but that does not have the profound impact that holding, stroking, and physically calming your loved one has.

Many couples begin their relationship with a lot of touching and nonsexual contact, but often this contact stops after a while. Once their couplehood is established, their touching becomes limited, occurring mostly or only during sexual contact. If there is one specific complaint I hear more than any other it is, "Whenever he (or she) touches me it always has to lead to sex." When touch becomes one-dimensional, or limited to a particular context, it affects the emotional tenor of the relationship.

So why do we need exercises? Many skeptics think that an "exercise" for emotional intimacy is a gimmick, that intimacy just naturally happens with physical closeness over time and that you can't do anything to hasten or improve it. I disagree, and so would the many couples with whom I have worked. These exercises are conscious ways to introduce the behavior that makes for intimate loving. They are not gimmicks if they are done from the heart, with honest openness, with the loving mindset, and without manipulative intent. An emotional bond cannot be forced, but it needs to be given the opportunity to grow. These exercises provide a nonsexual, nonverbal space for intimate feelings to be recognized and shared with each other. They start from your existing level of intimacy and, with the poetic nature of nonverbal communication, they deepen it.

All of the exercises in this chapter can be done by individuals who are just getting to know each other, couples who have been dating and sexually intimate for some time, and couples who have been married for years. They are perfect for couples who want to move gradually toward physical intimacy because all of these exercises are done fully clothed.

♀ Exercise ♂
Spoon Breathing

The first bonding exercise we will talk about is spoon breathing. Lie together on a bed or comfortable couch with one person's back snuggled up against the other person's front. You and your partner may already naturally fall into some form of this embrace—a lot of couples do—but don't wait for it to happen spontaneously. It's okay to ask your partner, "Can we spoon for a while?"

The Exercise   Lie on your sides with your legs bent so that you fit together like two spoons in a drawer. If you have a back problem and use a pillow support, have your partner snuggle up around the pillow as close as possible. The person who is in back can wrap an arm around the person in front, or just rest a hand on his or her stomach or side if a tight embrace is uncomfortable. Ask your partner her or his level of comfort, and respect what they say. Once you are snuggled together, lie still, letting go of any tensions, and try not to talk or squirm. Pay attention to your own breathing and to your partner's breathing.

Slow your breathing down by taking three or four deep breaths and exhaling forcefully. Make sure that all your muscles are relaxed. Concentrate on each leg individually and imagine that it is sinking into the bed. Picture your shoulders sinking into the bed. Pay attention to the overall sensations of warmth and closeness that wash over you and your partner as you lie together.

You may notice as you spoon breathe for a few minutes that both of you will relax and begin breathing in sync with each other.

You can spoon breathe at any time and in a variety of ways: clothed or in the nude, in the morning before getting up or in the evening to unwind after work. If you are uncomfortable in your relationship or are in a new relationship, begin spooning fully clothed. If you and your partner aren't comfortable being nude around each other, you can begin at night, in bed, with the lights off. Eventually you may enjoy spooning naked, in low lights. A lot of couples like to fall asleep in the spoon position. I encourage couples to spoon for at least ten minutes a day, either upon waking in the morning or when winding down at night before bed.

♀ Exercise ♂
Eye Gazing

Here is a bonding exercise I think you will find more intimate than spoon breathing. It is said that the eyes are windows to the soul, and I believe it. Gazing deeply into our lover's eyes can stop time. It makes us aware of who we are and brings that right up front to our partners, releasing modesty or defensiveness. In a gaze we recognize new, unknown aspects of our lover. We connect with the familiar in each other and welcome the undiscovered. As our eyes focus, our hearts open.

Remember that one of the two aspects of a relationship that differentiates couples who are truly in love from couples who simply like each other is the time spent gazing into each other's eyes. (And the other aspect? The amount of time they spend touching, of course!)

The Exercise Lie together on your bed, or sit comfortably, and face each other. Wrap your arms loosely around each other, or rest your hands in your partner's hands (you can take turns doing this), and gaze into each other's eyes for several minutes without talking.

Maybe you two used to do this when you first met. Remember how good it felt? Enjoy the feelings that come up for you now. How have they grown richer with time?

You can repeat this exercise every now and again when you feel a need or a desire to reconnect with each other. So often couples talk at each other or to each other, but they neglect to take the time to slow down and *be with* the other.

There may be times when you want to Eye Gaze and be consciously aware of the feelings that come up in you. This kind of eye gazing can be an internal barometer, telling you where you are in your relationship with your lover. When do you feel shy, or when does your lover seem shy? Do you feel exposed, or open? Do you want to talk or to just "be" together? Can you see current events and energy levels reflected in your partner's eyes, or do you feel them in your own? Over time you and your partner will rediscover the richness of your unspoken communication and the vocabulary your eyes speak only to each other.

♀ Exercise ♂
The Nurturing Lover

A simple part of being lovers is to care for each other's well-being. Too often we forget that it is okay to care for our loved one and that it is also okay for her or him to care for us. In fact, nurturing each other is an important facet of intimate relationships. If you have had a bad day, or if you both need some downtime together, have your partner nurture you.

The Exercise You can nurture just about anywhere: in bed, on the couch, or on the floor leaning against the couch. One person sits with his back against the wall or a support while the other lies with her head on that person's chest, in whatever way is comfortable. Then the person behind tenderly wraps his arms around the person in front.

Share this embrace for ten minutes. Close your eyes. Listen to each other's breathing. Feel each other's warmth. Feel your hearts beat.

If you have back problems or other physical issues, make sure when nurturing—and in all the other exercises in this book—that you have the proper supports you need to be really comfortable. Intimacy isn't much fun if you are in pain, or anxious because your partner's weight is pressing on an old injury. You may find it most comfortable to sit in a chair and have your partner sit between your legs. From there you can stroke his or her shoulders, neck, face and hair, while "holding" your partner gently between your legs. When you are being nurtured, you might be most comfortable resting your head on a pillow in your partner's lap, or using a pillow support between your knees. When nurturing each other it's important that you do whatever you need to do to make both of you feel physically comfortable and "taken care of."

♀ Exercise ♂
The Supportive Lover

How much of your partner have you ever felt at one time? Have you ever carried your partner, or vice versa? So often we support each other emotionally, but we rarely explore what is it like to support each other in other ways.

This is a good exercise for the evening, when you are winding down, or after a workout, when your breathing is strong and your energy is in balance. It is not recommended that you do this after dinner when your stomach is full.

The Exercise Lie on your back on your bed and have your partner slowly lower himself or herself on top of you, from toes to nose. The person on top should gradually allow his or her full weight to be supported by the person on the bottom. Move your heads around until you find a comfortable connection. Lie together quietly for several minutes. Depending on what is comfortable for the two of you, lie together nude or clothed, or under the covers.

Although the idea of doing this might make you anxious, this position is surprisingly possible and comfortable for most people. It does not seem to make much of a difference if one person is much larger than the other, since your weight spreads out over a larger area (and the bed). Move around until you find a position that works. If one of you is taller than the other, for example, you can lie so that your faces are close together and your feet farther apart. If one of you is much heavier than the other, place pillows or bolsters next to your partner's shoulders and under yours, so that your weight rests partially on the pillows and partially on your partner.

After trying this a couple times move around to find a position that you enjoy. Many people enjoy having their faces very close; others enjoy hearing and feeling their partner's heartbeat on their cheek.

If you have a back problem that prevents you from lying flat comfortably, skip this exercise. Instead, be creative about finding ways to "take the weight" of your partner. For example, as your partner sits next to you on the couch, or in a chair across from you, take his or her feet in your lap, hold them and warm them with your hand. Feel the weight of this often neglected, hard working part of the body, and nurture it.

♀ Exercise ♂
Palm Energy

This is a wonderful way to become aware of the intangible energy of your relationship. Sit cross-legged facing each other. Gaze lovingly into each other's eyes and do not waver. Just as your arms can embrace each other's bodies, can your gaze caress each other's souls?

The Exercise   Raise your hands and place your palms up against each other (as if you were playing a child's "patty-cake" game). Hold them there for ten seconds. Feel the heat running between you. Now slowly move your hands apart so that they no longer touch but are just close enough so that you can feel a current of energy flow between you. Concentrate on that flow for five minutes.

♀ Exercise ♂
Couple Rituals

Most of us have little rituals that we perform every day, both individually and, if we are in relationships, as couples. It doesn't matter what age we are, what culture we live in, or how conventional or liberated we think we are—we all ritualize many activities during the day, from how and where we shave or shower, to which club, bar, or coffee shop we go to regularly, to which television program we always watch. Rituals are a way of structuring time, of finding the familiar in the empty space of every day.

Something you can do to bond better right from the beginning of a relationship, or any time during one, is to start your own couple rituals. Couple rituals are things that you make a commitment to do with each other every day, week, or month. To the natural individual tendency to ritualize they add the couple dimensions of mutuality and commitment. You can use them to celebrate each other and the unique aspects of your relationship. This is especially important for people embarking on new relationships after the breakup of a long-term relationship or marriage, where there may be a tendency to unconsciously duplicate rituals from the prior relationship. It can also help those seeking to reinvent their current relationship and find new ways to bring meaning and pleasure to the time they already spend together.

By having rituals together you honor the importance of your relationship. Too often people take their partners for granted. So, your purpose and intention when setting up a ritual is key. You and your partner should feel one hundred percent focused on the activity and on each other. At the same time, these activities should be things you enjoy together. They are commitments, not chores.

With rituals you can make the familiar unfamiliar and the mundane special. Here are examples of rituals that have been shared by couples I know.

Bonding Breakfasts   Once a week get up a half-hour earlier and have coffee or breakfast together. Don't read the paper and don't talk about work problems, just focus on catching up with each other. Or take turns bringing the breakfast to bed.

A Gentle Garden   If you garden, plant a special area together with something beautiful or bountiful, and tend it together.

Romantic Dinners   Take turns cooking for each other, or cook meals together on a regular basis. If you have kids at home, this is a dinner for two, not for the whole family. If this won't work at home for you, dine out.

"How Do I Love Thee? Let Me Count the Ways..."   Spend an evening every so often reading favorite books or poems aloud. Alternate who reads and who listens. Read in nature, read by candlelight, go on road trips and read in the car or a camper, rent a canoe and read in the middle of a lake . . .

Virtual Vacations   Once a month, pretend you are visitors in your own town, and spend a day sightseeing—visit museums and historical places, hang out at the tourist "traps," go to the theater, whatever. Alternate who chooses the itinerary if you tend to enjoy different things!

Tango for Two   Take ballroom dancing lessons (or disco, or jazz, or salsa . . .), and then go out dancing on a regular basis.

A Time to Worship   If you are religious, attend a worship service together on a regular basis. Hold hands during parts of the worship when you are especially moved or inspired. Imagine you are singing some of the hymns for your partner. Close your eyes and try to feel the divine love or the eternal spirit that flows through your partner.

The key to couple rituals is not what you agree to do together, it is that you commit to doing it regularly, that you both participate mutually, and that you both look forward to it. Your ritual could even be an agreement to talk about a particular subject at a particular time: the kids or grandchildren, your financial situation, an upcoming vacation, or things you think would improve your relationship. These are all rituals that have been successful for many couples.

If you decide to have a conversation as part of your ritual commitment to each other, that conversation should be guided by love. For example, discussions about your financial situation or childrearing could easily lead to blaming and conflict. You must agree to discuss the issue at hand with a positive spin, in the context of how it strengthens or weakens your relationship as a couple and what you as a couple can do about the situation.

* * *

Lovemaking starts before you reach the bedroom, and continues long after you leave it. If you think of everything you do together as adding dimensions to your emotional bond, you will discover new depths for both yourself and your relationship.

Chapter 3
The Loving Touch

I n this chapter I hope to convince you that touch is a vital part of your relationship with your partner. Our touch can convey a number of things nonverbally, and there are many different ways to touch. There is a particular type of touch, called sensate focus touch, which best conveys love, whether it is self-love or the love you want to express to your partner when you make love. This is the style of touch that you will learn in the rest of this chapter.

Different people respond to being touched in different ways. By paying attention to your partner's responses and being aware of his or her physical uniqueness, you will discover that as a couple you have your own rhythms of pleasure and touch.

After many years of being together, you and your partner may have fallen into certain habitual ways of touching each other, both sexually and nonsexually. The sensate focus exercises in this chapter will give you a fresh perspective on what touch is all about, and help you look at the touch patterns in your relationship so that you can enhance the good ones, change the not-so-good ones, and reintroduce spontaneity.

For those of you in new relationships, as your physical intimacy develops you need to be careful about not automatically transferring the touch patterns of your previous relationship. Again, sensate focus exercises will give you a new dimension to explore in your physical intimacy.

The Essence of Touch

The essence of touch begins with our skin. We may not realize it, but many of us have never learned to show love for our own body through how we touch it. Beginning in childhood, society bombards us with unrealistic messages about what our body is and what it should be. We soon lose the immediate connection we have with our bodies as infants, and learn to mistrust or suppress the naturally sensuous pleasure we get from it. Many of us acquire negative images about our bodies or feel guilty about touching ourselves sensually—anywhere. At the very least we grow up detached from our bodies, viewing them as garments or tools. We forget that accepting our body allows us to open up to the full pleasure it is capable of. Only then are we able to share that pleasure with another.

Making love reconnects our mind and body and uses the power of that unity for our health and well-being. If improving our ability to use our body to convey love is what we are after, how our body *feels* is more important than what it *does* or how it *looks*. The key to knowing our body's feelings lies in the simple ability to give and receive touch.

Ultimately, touch is the spark that fires our passion. It is the basic medium through which we express and receive the joy we feel when we make love.

Touch Is Vital

Much research has been done on the critical nature of touch. Through decades of study of humans, primates, and other animals, researchers have discovered that touch is necessary for newborns of all species to survive and thrive. In his classic book *Touching*, Ashley Montagu describes how skin-to-skin contact affects our mental and physical health through all stages of our lives, beginning with birth and infancy.

As infants we need to be stroked, held, rocked, and cuddled to become physically healthy children and emotionally healthy adults. As adults, touch lowers our heart rate and blood pressure, promotes physical relaxation, and gives us feelings of general well-being. For people facing medical recovery, touch is extra important. Many studies have shown that patients touched by nurses recover faster than those who are not. Regardless of the hows and whys uncovered by scientific research, the bottom line is that touch is vital. The countless good ways that touch benefits us may be the reason we feel so good when touched.

Touching also makes it easier to share feelings. Studies show that touch brings us closer together, and encourages intimacy on multiple levels. Touch also encourages self-disclosure. It appears that being touched in intimate areas taps into intimate thoughts and feelings. Studies show that patients touched in the genital region by doctors and nurses during a physical examination often reveal personal sexual information. If touch can foster such openness during a professional medical encounter, imagine what it can do in the context of a loving relationship.

The Power of Touch

Touch carries great nonverbal power. Next to facial expression, touch is probably the best communicator of how we feel, since nonverbal communication tends to be less censored than verbal communication. In the language of nonverbal communication, touch is an "intensifier." This means that touch will make whatever mood already exists in a given situation stronger.

Not all touch intensifies *good* feelings. Let's say you have just met someone and, for whatever reason, this person gives you the creeps. If he or she then touches you, your feelings toward him or her will become even more negative.

Remember the first time you and your partner touched before you became lovers? Who touched first, or was it mutual? Think about whether that pattern of touch set the course for how your relationship unfolded.

Now that your relationship is established, are you aware of the subtleties of the way you touch? For example, does one of you always bend at the knees or stand on tiptoes when hugging or kissing? Do you put your arms over or under your partner's when you hug? Who initiates most of your touch? These are typical unconscious patterns we tend to fall into. See what happens when you change them, shake them up a bit. Maybe it feels physically awkward at first—or maybe it slightly changes the tone and tenor of the way you relate on a fundamental level.

Benefits of Touch

There are specific benefits to touch—besides the obvious!—that can help you make love better. First, touch is highly relaxing, and relaxation is a necessary state in which to begin making love. Second, touch can convey positive expectations. It can intensify an already positive situation (such as lovemaking). Third, touch can contribute to our sense of well-being. And most importantly, touch can convey love to our partner.

A sexual, intimate relationship offers an excellent context in which we can experience the loving power of touch. Sadly, the social norms for adults in North American culture do not encourage or allow much physical contact. For many of us, especially men, sexual encounters are the only situations in which we actively touch other human beings and enjoy being touched by them.

The Loving Touch

There are a number of different types of touch: the companionate touch of a friend, the nurturing touch of a parent, the rejuvenating touch of a healer, the arousing sexual touch of a lover, the energetic touch of massage, and so forth. We are all capable of giving and receiving a broad spectrum of touch.

Just as there are different types of touch, there are different ways to touch. The first step in making love better than ever is to learn a particular kind of touch—and way to touch—which conveys love. This type of loving touch is called *sensate focus* touch, and is a core element in the exercises you will learn in this book.

Sensate focus touch was pioneered by the well-known sex therapists Masters and Johnson to treat couples with sexual problems. Having used sensate focus technique over many years, I have found that it is the best way to convey love to your partner through touch, especially when you combine it with the loving mindset you read about in Chapter 1.

The term sensate focus may sound technical but it is actually quite simple and self-explanatory. Sensate focus is a technique in which you *focus* your attention as closely as you can on the *sensations* in your skin. This is the key to all of the exercises in this book: direct all your attention—and intention—on where you touch your skin, or your partner's skin, and where your partner touches you. Don't think about how you were just touching, or how you should touch next. Don't think about "the next step." If your mind wanders off at any point during an exercise, consciously bring it back to the place of your connection and what you are experiencing, to the moment you are in and the sensations you feel.

This sensate focus touch is called a *caress*. It is a delicate but definite touch to the skin. It is not a massage, rubbing, or pressure stroke, and it isn't a tentative, soft, brushing glide either. A loving sensate focus caress has the following characteristics:

It is very slow. As you caress during the exercises in the book, practice slowing the speed at which you touch by half whenever you think of it.

It is pressure-free. There should be no pressure for you or your partner to perform sexually. (I'll say more about this in Chapter 6.)

It is focused. Pay attention to the temperature, texture, contrast, and shape of what you touch. If you become distracted at any point, consciously bring your mind back to the point of touch.

It is in the here and now. As you touch, if you start thinking about the past or the future, bring yourself back to what you feel now.

It is sensuous and sensual. As you touch, experience the pure pleasure of your skin on your partner's skin.

The three exercises that follow will introduce you to sensate focus touch. If you find these unusual at first, or feel awkward or self-conscious, take your time with them. Don't rush through them, but repeat them at your own speed until you become comfortable with this kind of conscious touching.

♀ Exercise ♂
Touching an Object

In this first exercise, you will touch an inanimate object. It may seem a little silly at first, but I have asked you to begin with an object, not with yourself or your lover, so that you are not as self-conscious. This will give you the opportunity to practice sensate focus techniques without having to worry about conveying the intention of sexual loving. By the time you do come together with your partner, touching in this loving way will be second nature.

Before You Begin Set aside about fifteen minutes during which you will not be disturbed. Pick two or three objects that feel good to the touch, such as a piece of velvet, a peach, and a smooth, odd-shaped stone.

The Exercise Place one of the items in your lap and lightly touch it with rhythmic strokes as slowly as you can. Close your eyes. Focus all of your attention on how your fingers feel and what they feel. Don't think about something that just happened or what is to come; simply be in the present.

Caress the object in different ways—stroking with the nap, against the nap, in a circular motion, up and down. Explore the shape and surface of the object with your fingertips.

If your mind drifts off, bring it back to what you are doing. Get in touch with your sensuality—how this object feels against your skin.

Caress very slowly. If you think you are already moving your hand slowly, try cutting your speed in half and see how this affects your ability to focus.

Next, pick up the second item and begin again.

Stop the exercise after fifteen minutes. Can you feel how relaxed and focused you became from this simple act of touching? Your breathing has slowed and your heart rate has slowed. This simple touching exercise has the same effect as meditation. It harmonizes or unifies your mind, your body, and your feelings.

♀ Exercise ♂
Touching Yourself

In this exercise you will learn how you would like to be touched by trying some sensate focus caresses on yourself. Remember, though, the emphasis of a loving touch is *sensual*, not *sexual*. By learning to touch yourself in a relaxing, gentle, and loving way you will learn how to give and receive loving touch.

Do you feel self-conscious caressing yourself? Many people do, especially when they move to sensitive areas like their genitals and especially if they have never touched themselves in this way before. This feeling is natural, but will fade as you practice. It is very important to learn about your own body responses so that you can increase your ability to become aroused and awaken your ability to love yourself and your partner. Of course, as with any exercise, don't do anything that makes you uncomfortable or that feels threatening. Go at your own pace.

The Exercise   Choose a setting where you have privacy and will not be disturbed. Pick a small area of your body—your arm, chest, or thigh—for your first self-caress. Put a little lotion or massage oil on your fingertips and slowly begin to touch this area of your body.

Touch gently and focus on the different sensations you feel. Focus on the exact point of contact between your hand and your body. If your mind wanders off to something else, bring it back to exactly how your skin feels, both your fingertips and the part being touched. Stroke yourself slowly and lightly. Touch only the skin; do not press hard or try to massage your muscles. Can you feel the contours of your body? The individual hairs on your skin?

Think about what you feel right now rather than anything you have been taught or remember from the past. If you have trouble concentrating, slow down your touch. Use more lotion if your skin feels rough or dry.

Spend fifteen minutes or so learning the feeling of your touch against your skin.

♀ Exercise ♂
Touching Your Pleasure Centers

In this exercise you will use the loving touch to caress your genitals, but this touch is not masturbation. Many adults use masturbation as a comforting way to receive touch, but the genital caress is different. The goal of this touch is not to feel sexual, turn yourself on, or come to climax. The goal is to learn what kinds of touch you can feel in your genitals and what feels good. If you do the exercise with the loving mindset I talked about in Chapter 1, you will also learn that it is loving—not selfish—to touch yourself.

Before You Begin   If you live with children make sure you will not be disturbed, and secure your privacy. Sit or lie naked in a comfortable position, in a comfortable space. If you are not used to being naked openly, lie or recline in bed under light covers. Remember that caressing is not the same as masturbating. Reassure yourself that you are not doing anything wrong; you are learning to enhance your ability to share pleasure with your partner. The purpose of this exercise is not to have an orgasm but to learn the different pleasurable sensations of your body.

The Exercise for Women   Warm a little baby oil or other lubricant on your fingers and begin to slowly touch your inner thighs and your vaginal lips. If any part of your body feels tense, slow down, and make a conscious effort to relax it. During this caress you may include only your thighs, or your outer genitalia, or stroke inside your vagina as well. Do whatever you are comfortable with and will enjoy.

Concentrate on the touch exactly the way you did when you caressed the other part of your body in the previous exercise. Focus on the warmth, texture, and contours of your touch. If your mind starts to wander off, slow down the movement of your hand and consciously bring your mind back to that point where skin touches skin.

Try different touches. Touch yourself the way your partner usually touches you, then the way you usually touch yourself, then try a completely different way. Do not spend any more time on the clitoris than you do on other parts of your genitals. Pay attention to the landscape of your body—the changes in texture, temperature, and arousal as you touch different areas.

If you do become sexually aroused don't worry, but remember that it is not your goal. The only goals are to enjoy yourself and to learn about your own body. If you become tense, make a conscious effort to relax your muscles and take a deep breath. Gently, slowly stroke yourself to feel maximum sensual awareness and enjoyment. If you have an orgasm, that is okay. Don't try to make it happen and don't try to push it away. Just experience it.

The Exercise for Men   Warm some baby oil or lotion on your fingers if you like, or just make sure your hands are warm. Slowly begin to caress your penis and scrotum, concentrating on the temperature and texture of your skin. Don't worry about whether or not you have an erection—it is not important to the exercise. You are just exploring the sensations your penis and scrotum are capable of and which types of touch feel good.

Keep your attention on the exact point of contact between your fingers and your genitals. If your mind wanders off, slow the movement of your hand and bring your mind back to the touch. Experiment with different types of touch. Touch yourself the way you usually do, the way your partner does, and in as many different ways as you can think of.

Keep all the muscles in your body relaxed and breathe evenly. If you feel yourself approaching ejaculation, that is okay. Don't push to make it happen, try to make it better, or push it away. Slow down your touch, breathe deeply, and relax. If you have an erection and feel yourself losing it, don't panic. You're just exploring, and you can always find your way back here again. Continue caressing for fifteen minutes.

•   •   •

These three simple exercises are the key to enhancing your sensual vocabulary. You may be impatient to start with the partner exercises—after all this is a book about making love—but I encourage you to spend time with these exercises till you feel really comfortable doing them. You will learn some really important things about what feels sensual to you, how you like to be touched, and your capacity to feel arousal. In the next chapter we will explore how to increase your capacity for arousal, and increase your awareness of it. Becoming more aware of your own arousal patterns will help you become more sensitive to the changes that take place in your partner's body and mind as he or she becomes aroused.

Chapter 4
Loving Yourself

Have you ever heard the saying, "You can't love another person unless you love yourself"? Most people interpret that saying to mean that you can't love another person unless you respect yourself enough to keep away from self-destructive habits or think highly enough of yourself that you pamper yourself. I also extend this to our sexual nature—you can't make love to another person unless you can convey love to yourself through your touch. This chapter will show you how.

Do you think of masturbation as self-love? Many people do. It always amazed me when I looked up "masturbation" in the dictionary when I was a child that it was either defined as "self-abuse" or "self-pollution"! As a sex therapist, listening to some people describe the way they masturbate or watching them masturbate, I have lamented that it really *was* self-abuse. Some people literally flog and beat their genitals in order to become sexually aroused. To me this is the antithesis of self-love. Loving yourself means treating all of your body, and *especially* your genitals and erogenous zones, with respect. It means touching yourself in a way that conveys that you love yourself. It means recognizing that your body is a gift, a remarkable, sensitive, and complex instrument of feeling and the container of your life energies that is, in the truest sense, your spirit's home. It deserves respect and love, and in return it will give you health and pleasure.

Loving yourself means being able to open yourself up fully to sexual experience, and the emotions and physical responses that can entail. While this sounds self-evident, for many people it is not. Beginning in childhood, we have developed hundreds of ways to contain or suppress our emotions and our arousal. We are told not to cry—which is an arousal reaction—after upsetting experiences. We are told not to laugh or to shout when excited. When men hit puberty they learn to control their spontaneous erections. Women learn to hide whether a boy turns them on, and they learn how to respond to a boy in ways that give the "right," not the "wrong" impression.

In a good sexual loving relationship, room has to be made to experience and express more of this arousal. We need to release ourselves from the behavioral patterns that inhibit or distort our passion and emotion, and the sexual response that results from them. Without this, sexual expression is not fully balanced, and cannot tap the rich depths of what it means to share sexual loving.

Sexual Fitness

Loving yourself also means developing your sexual fitness. One of the important aspects of good sexual loving is deepening your capacity for sexual arousal. Like fitness training, which you do to get your body into peak athletic condition, sexual fitness exercises get your body in peak sexual shape, so you are physically able to experience the best sexual arousal. Do you find it strange that you can train for love as you might train for athletics? It isn't. You can't separate your body from your mind and your psyche. If you want to experience enhanced loving in your psyche and soul, you have to get your body ready to go along. Your body provides the energy to do it with. First, let me explain a few things about physiology and the sexual response.

Mastering Your Ability to Relax

In order to make love and experience your entire range of sexual arousal you need to begin with a state of relaxation. This sounds contrary to what most people think. "Wait a minute!" they say, "When I make love I'm excited!" Actually, as you make love, you *become* excited. And the more relaxed you are when you start, the more excited you will get. This has to do with the way our nervous system is built.

The nervous system is the wiring that allows different parts of the body to communicate with each other. It includes the brain and the spinal cord, as well as all of the peripheral nerves that branch off from the spinal cord. These peripheral nerves either control voluntary muscles, or they are part of the network of nerves that controls automatic responses such as heartbeat and digestion. We generally think of these autonomic processes as body functions that we do not have control over.

The autonomic nervous system has two separate and complementary parts—the sympathetic nervous system and the parasympathetic nervous system. The sympathetic nervous system delivers the so-called "fight or flight" response, and speeds up your physical responses. It floods you with adrenaline so that you can fight, run away, or otherwise deal with a threatening event. When this system is active you experience a combination of physical signs: your heart beats rapidly, your eyes dilate, you perspire, and blood rushes away from the center of your body to your limbs. If these physical responses occur in reaction to something that is not a threatening event, you experience *anxiety*.

The parasympathetic nervous system is just the opposite. It is active when your body takes care of its life-sustaining processes, such as regulating heartbeat and digestion. It slows your body down so that you conserve energy. As a result, we experience this system's activity as relaxation.

So what is the tie-in to making love, you ask? The sympathetic and parasympathetic systems generally cannot be active at the same time. We know this from first-hand experience because it is difficult to be relaxed when we are anxious or aroused. Sexual activity is the only situation I know of in which these two systems work together, rather than antagonistically. And to make satisfying, full-spectrum love, you need to be able to cultivate sensual arousal while consciously engaging your relaxation nervous system.

When you activate your relaxation response and then begin stimulation, your capacity for arousal and pleasure increases. As you become more aroused, your energetic sympathetic nervous system comes into play, causing your heart rate, blood pressure, and breathing to increase. Your relaxation response peaks right before orgasm, which is a parasympathetic response that causes an instantaneous return to the relaxed state. What a beautiful system! What it means, though, is that your sexual response will function best if you learn to relax yourself. That is what the next two exercises will show you.

♀ Exercise ♂
Belly Breathing

Proper breathing is the basis of life—and of feeling alive. The oxygen we take in with every breath is our lifeline, but a lot of us don't breathe properly, and the way we breathe can create or exacerbate sexual problems. If we are anxious or nervous, our breathing becomes constricted and we take in less oxygen. The first step in becoming sexually fit is to breathe in a way that relaxes you and nourishes you with oxygen.

The Exercise Lie comfortably on your back on your bed, or recline in a supportive chair. Loosen any tight clothing. Place one hand on your abdomen and the other on your heart. Now take a deep, slow breath that you can feel all the way down to your abdomen. Breathe as if you are drawing breath down through your body, into your legs and toes. This type of breath should cause your abdomen to expand and rise; when you exhale, it should contract.

As you breathe, inhaling and exhaling should be one continuous process. Don't hold your breath after you inhale but let it flow. Feel the air flowing all the way into your lungs and your belly, and all the way out. Visualize that air as a white light flowing in and out of you, not only relaxing you but also energizing you. If you want to, rest after each exhalation.

It may take time to get over the feeling of "forcing" your breath into this pattern; that is because you are engaging your conscious mind into your autonomic function. With just a little practice it will become natural and comfortable—you will have developed the ability to consciously engage your autonomic systems. Notice how your body has its own rhythms?

Once you have learned to breathe like this, spend some time "belly breathing" each day. Take two deep belly breaths and then breathe normally for about a minute. Take two belly breaths again and breathe normally for another minute. Breathe in this pattern for about ten minutes, and you may just find you are more relaxed—and ener-gized—throughout your day.

♀ Exercise ♂
Deep Muscle Relaxation

This is another exercise to help you learn how to use your mind to engage—or disengage! —your muscles. It is a great exercise to use any time you feel overly anxious, stressed, or are unwinding before falling asleep.

The Exercise Lie on your back on your bed, or sit reclining in a comfortable chair. Starting with your large muscle groups, tighten each group of muscles in your body from your feet up—legs, torso, arms, face and head—and hold them as tight as you can for a couple of seconds, then release them. Try to breathe deeply and evenly as you do this exercise.

After you have tried this exercise a couple of times, and feel you have gotten it down, try isolating your muscle groups even more: tense just your feet muscles, then just your calves, just your thighs, and so forth. When you feel very advanced, work your way up your body as usual, then when you reach your face and head work your way back down to your toes again.

As a bonding variation, you can talk your partner through this relaxation process, then have him or her do the same for you. If your partner falls asleep before the end of the exercise, that is okay. Put a blanket over your partner and let him or her doze. The sleep that comes from this is usually restful and energizing.

♀ Exercise ♂
Body Image

Besides learning relaxation, to touch yourself in a loving way you will need to love your body—and that means loving the way it looks. For many people this is difficult. Our culture bombards us daily with messages that try to convince us that our looks are inadequate. The good news is that the touching exercises that you and your partner will learn in this book will help you love your body. After all, how could you not love something that gives you so much pleasure?

The first step to loving the way your body looks is to become comfortable with your looks. This body image exercise will help you.

Choose a time when you will not be disturbed and secure your privacy. First, take off all of your clothes and stand naked in front of a full-length mirror. Make sure that there is plenty of light in the room. Now gaze at your body. Take a few minutes to check out each part of yourself. Look with honest eyes, try to put aside your preconceptions and insecurities.

The Exercise: Part I   Begin with your face first and look into your eyes. Smile, and look at your mouth. Slowly move your gaze down, appreciating your shoulders, torso, arms and hands, on down to your feet. Then turn around and use a hand mirror so that you can look at the back of your body. Start with your hair, and work your way down to your ankles and heels. Take your time, and breathe and relax as you do this.

In addition to just looking and becoming comfortable with your body, mentally catalogue what you see. Talk to yourself and describe the different parts of your body—both positive and negative. Think about how each part of your body feels, how it sustains you, and how much pleasure it has brought you in the past. To finish the exercise lie down and do some belly breathing and some deep muscle relaxation.

Body Image: Part II   Try this exercise a week or two later and, as you look in the mirror and appreciate each part of your body, try and feel it from the inside at the same time. Are there parts of your body that you have difficulty feeling? These are parts from which you are more cut off, and you may have difficulty accepting loving touch to them and feeling arousal in them. You might want to spend some time thinking about why this may be, or you might want to spend more time touching and appreciating that part of your body.

Exercising Your Pelvic Muscles

In addition to knowing how to relax, it is important that certain muscles in your pelvic area are in good working order. Most of us acknowledge the importance of maintaining physical fitness but neglect our pelvic muscles. More muscle mass in the pelvis means that more blood can flow to the area when you become aroused. And this means more pleasure!

♀ Exercise ♂
PC Muscle for Women

Do you know what your PC muscle is, and where it is located? It is a muscle that runs along the floor of your pelvis, cradling your internal organs. It is the muscle that contracts when you start and stop your urine flow. It is the muscle that squeezes when you draw your vagina up and in.

Before You Begin   If you are unfamiliar with the PC muscle, first locate it. Place one of your fingers lightly against your vaginal lips or inside your vagina up to the first knuckle. Pretend you are urinating and you want to stop the flow. The muscle that tightens around your finger when you do this is the PC muscle group. Internally you should feel a drawing together or a drawing upward in your vaginal and pelvic area. Once you have located the muscle there is no need to keep your hand on it as you tighten and relax it.

As you do the following exercise, be careful not to tense your abdomen or thigh muscles when you are squeezing your PC. Keep your breathing relaxed and steady. You should be able to tighten your PC muscle without anyone looking at you being able to tell that you are doing so.

The Exercise   Three times a day spend a few minutes flexing and relaxing your PC muscle. Start with three to five repetitions and build to more as you feel comfortable. It is better to do five repetitions three times a day than to do twenty repetitions only once a day. The PC muscle tires easily and may not relax fully each time you flex when you first start, but it will tone up quickly.

If you get tired after three repetitions, stop. Without use, this muscle gets untrained and it takes time to build it back up again. Also, this muscle spasms very easily, so you don't want to push it too hard. Spasms are counterproductive to mastering the squeeze. To avoid them, try to consciously feel your PC muscle relaxing after each squeeze, and don't squeeze again until you feel it is totally relaxed.

Keep in mind that you can do these flexes anytime and anywhere, even while waiting at a stoplight, since they are not apparent to anyone but you. After a while you might want to practice doing the PC squeeze while doing something else, such as brushing your teeth.

These exercises were first developed by an obstetrician, Dr. A.H. Kegel, to control incontinence in pregnant women and women who had just given birth. That's why they are often referred to as Kegel exercises.

A strong PC muscle has many benefits for women. It tightens and tones the vagina, and gives you better bladder control. A strong PC muscle also makes it easier to have orgasms. In both men and women, flexing the PC muscle at the moment of orgasm intensifies the orgasm. This is because when your PC muscle is in shape, more blood can flow to and from the genital area. And aside from all of the reasons given above, doing this exercise is fun and feels good.

♀ Exercise ♂
PC Muscle for Men

Before You Begin   Your PC muscle is the muscle that runs along the floor of your pelvis, cradling your internal organs. To locate your PC muscle lightly place two fingers behind your testicles. Now imagine that you are urinating and want to stop the flow. The muscle that you squeeze internally to stop the flow is the PC muscle. When urinating, you can practice stopping and starting a couple of times so that you feel confident you are familiar with this muscle group.

The Exercise   Every day, three times a day, flex and relax this muscle group a few times. You can begin with three to five repetitions, and work your way up to whatever feels good. Be careful not to overdo this, however. You want to develop control, but you don't want to overdevelop the muscle. More than twenty repetitions at a time may cause your PC muscle to get sore. Men with prostate problems may find this muscle a bit harder to train; however, doing so will be rewarding and is beneficial to prostate health.

To do the PC Squeeze, isolate the muscle and relax your abdomen, buttocks, and all other muscles (including your facial muscles). Breathe evenly as you squeeze and relax. You may feel slightly aroused because when you exercise this muscle you are increasing blood flow into the genital area, but don't worry if you don't.

It will take about three weeks for your PC muscle to get in shape, and then you really need to do this exercise for the rest of your life. Men whose PC muscle is in good shape can have more enjoyable erections, more sensation in the genital area, better ejaculation control, stronger orgasms, and even multiple orgasms.

Improved prostate health is another important benefit of the PC muscle exercise for men. The stronger your PC muscle is, the stronger your ejaculations will be, which means that your prostate gland is more likely to expel all of its contents during ejaculation. Men who have consistent, complete ejaculations tend to have fewer problems with prostate enlargement.

♀ Exercise ♂
Advanced PC Muscle for Men and Women

After you have done the basic PC muscle exercise for six weeks or two months, try this advanced version. In addition to a set of quick repetitions add half as many slow repetitions. You should be able to feel your PC muscle slowly suck in and then slowly push back out. Try to gradually tense the muscle for five seconds, hold it for five seconds, and then push back out for five seconds. The first time you may only be able to do this once or twice. Eventually you can work up to ten repetitions. It may take you days or weeks—the time doesn't matter, the improved muscle tone does.

♀ Exercise ♂
Pelvic Tilts, Thrusts, and Rolls

This set of exercises—pelvic thrusts, rolls, and tilts—are for your abdomen, buttocks, and thigh muscles. They help loosen up and release the tension most people keep in these areas. If you work at a desk job or stand on your feet most of the day, you will find these exercises are very good for loosening up your hamstrings and the related pelvic muscle groups. They are equally good for both men and women.

Pelvic thrusts can be done either lying down or standing up (you can grasp the back of a chair for support, if you like). The idea is to rock your pelvis from back to front without moving any other parts of your body. It is especially important to keep from tensing your stomach or leg muscles.

Worried about back problems? In my experience most people can do pelvic thrusts, rolls, and tilts without risk, especially if they do them slowly and moderately. If you have back problems, go easy and consult your physician before attempting these exercises.

The Pelvic Thrust   If you are lying down, bring your knees up and place your feet flat on the bed. Lift your pelvis slowly up and down. This should be the only part of you that moves. Do it as quickly or as slowly as you like, and as many times as you like. You can rock to music if you wish, or vary the speed of your rocking.

The important things to focus on are keeping all your other muscles relaxed, and breathing deeply and evenly. Do not hold your breath. To make sure you are breathing correctly it may be helpful to exhale loudly or make a noise with each thrust.

To do pelvic thrusts while standing or walking, stand with your knees slightly bent and rock your pelvis back and forth. Or—for the more coordinated—as you walk, consciously thrust your pelvis forward with each step.

The Pelvic Roll   Pelvic rolls are similar to thrusts. These are easier to do standing up, but you can also do them lying down.

Roll your hips in a circular fashion backwards-sideways-forward-sideways in a continuous motion. Think of Elvis Presley. If you have difficulty getting the hang of this movement, or if you feel playful, buy a hula-hoop and practice with that. Practice rolls at different speeds, and practice rolling as slowly as you possibly can. Throughout, remember to relax the muscles in your buttocks, legs, and abdomen, and use your pelvic muscles to generate the movement. The secret to doing these exercises is to roll and thrust your pelvis while still staying loose.

To make this more enjoyable you can combine pelvic thrusts and rolls and do them to music. You should try to do a series of these thrusts and rolls for about ten minutes every day. Close your eyes so that you can really feel your body. Men, especially, tend to have tight hip muscles. Loosening them up can often increase your ability to become sexually aroused and have erections.

If you have a serious back problem, you might want to consider starting with the pelvic tilt (below), which is easier on the back. It should loosen tension and strengthen the muscles that support the lower back.

The Pelvic Tilt   Lie on your back with your knees up. Keep your lower back on the floor, and practice tilting your pelvis up and down. Bring your hips in toward your belly button and release them. This is similar to the pelvic thrust but your lower back stays on the floor and you have a smaller range of movement. Pelvic tilts can also be done standing up. Simply keep your lower back in the same position and tilt your pelvis back and forth.

. . .

A variety of types of physical exercises can be beneficial to lovemaking, especially anything that involves stretching, squatting, spreading your legs, and building strength in your legs. Aerobic activity is also great, not only for general cardiovascular benefits you're probably familiar with, but because it prompts relaxation, releases stress, and releases endorphins. If you keep your body's pleasure-releasing systems in shape your body will pay you back double by increasing the pleasure it experiences in other peak encounters—such as making love!

Chapter 5
Loving Arousal

Sexual arousal plays a fundamental role in making satisfying love. To make love better than ever you will need to broaden your understanding of sexual arousal and deepen your physical ability to experience sexual arousal. Sexual arousal is a complex response, drawing as it does on our mind, our emotions, and our bodies.

As we grow older, the way in which we experience and receive sexual pleasure may change. With age our emotional intelligence grows and our physical metabolism and hormones change, so it makes sense that our patterns of arousal should evolve, too. But many of us are unprepared for this change, and don't take advantage of it. Many people assume wrongly that sexual desire and sexual fulfillment decline with age. When physical and relationship changes begin to happen, they resign themselves to it. Others get frustrated when they find that the lovemaking "techniques" they used in the past don't work as well as they used to.

Making love better than ever means growing with these changes, being flexible and attentive to their sexual nuances. By doing so you and your partner can tap into the exciting new lovemaking that these changes can bring. Unleashing your full sexual potential as a couple means becoming familiar with your unique arousal patterns, deepening your capacity for arousal, and playing with or pushing your mutual arousal to the limits of what you and your partner want.

In this chapter (and this book) you will learn a lot about arousal awareness. As you go through the process of honing your arousal awareness process together, you may find that uncharted sexual territory opens up for you. Your sexual life may become less ordinary, more extraordinary. For new couples, this increases your chances of developing a sexual union that will deepen over time and not fall apart at the first sign of stress or boredom. For long-term couples, uncovering sexual newness can have a profound effect on other aspects of your overall relationship.

How Aroused Are You?

To get in touch with your arousal I will ask you to use a scale that I have adapted from the sensate focus approach. Think of your arousal as having three levels, which I will call *gentle, strong,* and *urgent.* "Gentle" can be considered the early stirrings of arousal, when you know you are aroused but don't feel you have to do anything more with it—when you enjoy the arousal just as it is. "Strong" is a more active, insistent arousal, when you feel you want to act further on the arousal, with a partner or alone. And "urgent" is the driving arousal that demands that you continue responding to it and can take you over the edge into orgasm.

The first exercise, Arousal Awareness, will familiarize you with this scale in terms of your own arousal. The Peaking and Plateauing exercises that follow will show you how understanding your arousal awareness will positively affect your lovemaking and sexual pleasure. Many of the exercises in this book draw on this arousal scale.

If you would like to work more with the sensate focus arousal scale, it forms the backbone of one of my other books, *Sexual Pleasure: Reaching New Heights of Arousal and Intimacy*. In that book you will find more detailed exercises that use a 1–10 scale for arousal awareness.

The Anatomy of Arousal

Did you find the anatomy lesson on relaxation in the last chapter helpful? Here is another brief one, explaining why sex is so pleasurable—and how it can be more so!

When we experience significant arousal or engage in strenuous physical activity our brain releases chemicals called *endorphins*. Endorphins are natural painkillers, with a chemical structure similar to that of heroin and other opiates. Scientists believe that the reason heroin and opiates have the effect they do is because our brain already contains receptors for them. Endorphins are also responsible for many of the euphoric mental states and altered states of consciousness we get from activities such as running and chanting.

Sexual arousal in particular causes us to release endorphins. And an intense orgasm can also cause a tremendous endorphin high. By building your sexual arousal in predictable ways, you release large amounts of endorphins over periods of time. This can feel great alone—which is where you will start—but with a partner it becomes an absolutely fantastic experience.

♀ Exercise ♂
Arousal Awareness

To develop arousal awareness we will begin to use the arousal scale explained above. Try to think of your sexual arousal as falling on a spectrum from "gentle" to "urgent," with "strong" arousal falling in between. The lower end of "gentle" is not being aroused at all, and the highest end of "urgent" is orgasm. "Gentle" includes mild twinges of arousal that come and go up to a constant low level of arousal. When you are strongly aroused, you feel that you would really like it to continue. When you reach urgent arousal, if you had to talk you would sound somewhat out of breath. The higher end of urgent arousal is the feeling that orgasm is inevitable.

The Exercise   Start with a genital caress on yourself. As you slowly stroke and explore your genitals, think of the different states of arousal you feel—gentle, strong, or urgent? Caress yourself for about twenty minutes and every five minutes or so ask yourself, "Where am I now?" Don't try to reach any particular level of arousal. In fact just notice how your arousal ebbs and flows. Focus, relax, and breathe. If you get distracted, bring your mind back to your touch.

Repeat this exercise until you are able to reliably experience "strong" arousal levels from this caress. Then try the next exercise.

For men, keep in mind that the level of your arousal is not necessarily related to how hard your erection is. Focus during the exercise on how aroused you feel and try to recognize your feelings of arousal internally without having to look at or feel your erection. For women, it is important to get in touch with the strengths and depths your arousal can reach. Remember that your arousal may not necessarily be reflected in the amount of your lubrication; this can fluctuate according to your menstrual cycles or the onset of menopause.

♀ Exercise ♂
Peaking

In this exercise you bring your arousal up to a peak, then let it subside, then bring it to another peak. This is the type of arousal pattern that releases maximum endorphins, increases your capacity for arousal, and builds your sexual energy.

The Exercise　To begin, relax, breathe, and caress your genitals as you did in the previous exercise. When you feel yourself reaching "strong" arousal, stop caressing and allow your arousal to go down to "gentle."

Then slowly begin caressing again. This time let yourself climb to a really strong level of arousal. Then stop and let your arousal subside again.

Caress yourself so that you reach very strong levels of arousal a couple times, if you can, and allow your arousal to go back down to gentle after each of these peaks. Continue this exercise for about twenty minutes or until you reach orgasm.

♀ Exercise ♂
Switching Focus by Yourself

There are a number of things you can focus on during sexual activity. A lot of people focus only on their genitals, but there is so much more. There are sights, smells, and sounds. Think of sex as a symphony. Most of us usually hear the composition as a whole, but if we slow down and pay closer attention, listen more carefully, we become able to pick out the different orchestra sections and even individual instruments.

Learning how to "listen to" or focus on both the orchestra and individual instruments during your lovemaking will open up new sexual pleasures and experiences for you and your partner. This exercise teaches you the technique of switching focus. Practice it first by yourself, then when you feel ready you can invite your partner to join in.

The Exercise To learn to switch focus lie comfortably on your bed or recline in a supportive chair, and begin to caress some part of your body—let us say it is your thigh. First become conscious of the feeling in your hand as it strokes your thigh; then switch to the feeling in your thigh as it is touched by your hand.

As you focus on sensations, see if you can switch your focus from your hand to your thigh and back again. This takes a little practice—don't expect to get it the first time around.

When you feel comfortable with this technique try using the technique during a genital caress. As you caress yourself, focus first on your hand touching your genitals, and then switch focus to your genitals being touched by your hand. Practice consciously switching your focus back and forth as you continue the genital caress for fifteen or twenty minutes. Do you notice changes in your arousal as you switch focus from one part of your body to another?

When doing the exercise with a partner, you can practice switching focus between the part of your body being caressed by your partner and a different part of your body that might be caressing your partner.

The next exercise, "Plateauing," will show you how to use this technique to deepen arousal.

♀ Exercise ♂
Plateauing

In the "Peaking" exercise you allowed your arousal to go up and down in a wave-like pattern. Plateauing is similar, but here you attempt to ride the crest of each arousal wave for a few seconds.

There are four techniques you can use to plateau: squeezing your PC muscle, deepening your breathing, changing your movements, and switching your focus. You can try this exercise on a couple of different occasions, each time using one of the techniques, or you can try combining a couple of techniques in one session. Practice these techniques till they become really familiar, and in future exercises you can use all of them without thinking about it.

Plateauing with Breaths   Begin doing a genital caress on yourself. When you reach a strong level of arousal, slow down your breathing and notice that you slide down to a gentler level of arousal. Keep caressing yourself so that your arousal doesn't drop too low, then speed up your breathing so that you climb to a very strong level or arousal. Repeat slowing and quickening your breath to regulate your levels of arousal. Eventually let yourself go all the way to climax.

Plateauing with the PC Squeeze   Repeat the pattern described above, but instead of changing your breathing, when you reach a fairly strong level of arousal give your PC muscle a quick squeeze. Your arousal level should drop as a result. Continue caressing until your arousal climbs back up to a strong level, and squeeze again. Do this once or twice more, or until you feel ready to climax. (Be careful not to do this too many times or to do squeezes too soon after each other, or you might arrest your arousal.)

Plateauing with Pelvic Thrusts   Begin a genital caress and do sensuous pelvic thrusts against your hand until you reach a strong level of arousal. At this point, stop thrusting and allow your arousal to drop somewhat. Then do pelvic thrusts again until you return to a strong level of arousal. Repeat the pattern a few times or until you feel like climaxing.

Plateauing by Shifting Your Focus   Begin a genital caress and continue caressing without stopping. This time when you reach a strong arousal level, shift your focus, so that although you are still touching yourself you are focusing on the feelings of another part of your body that you are not touching. Your arousal should slip down to a lower level. Now caress yourself again and see if you can reach an urgent arousal level.

Can you see how this works? By changing your breathing, flexing your PC muscle, varying your thrusting, and switching your focus, you are able to maintain your arousal at a particular level for anywhere from a few seconds up to a couple of minutes.

Taking Care of Yourself

Now that we have talked about specific relaxation exercises, pelvic exercises, and arousal exercises, let's talk for a minute about general health and fitness. A big part of loving yourself is staying healthy and refraining from self-destructive habits.

Are you in great physical condition—a triathlete or marathon runner? Or are you a fitness disaster area, a true couch potato? Most of us are somewhere in between. To develop your ability to experience arousal to your fullest potential you need to have a basic level of general fitness. What does this mean?

If you smoke, please do your best to stop now, or begin tapering off. It is a scientific fact that cigarette smoking is one of the worst things you can do for your love life. Nicotine is a stimulant that restricts blood flow to the small blood vessels in your skin. It erodes your ability to feel sensations and impairs circulation to the point that many smokers have difficulty having orgasms. For male smokers this includes difficulty getting and maintaining erections.

In addition to immediate benefits, don't you want to make sure that you are able to love your partner for a long, long time?

If you don't exercise on a regular basis, start simply. Start walking. Try to take a brisk walk for fifteen to twenty minutes every day. Any exercise you can get will energize you and prepare you for love-making. As always, you should consult your physician before you begin an exercise program.

Nutrition

I believe that eating and drinking, like making love, are among the greatest pleasures in life. Simple pleasures like these are largely the things in life that you share with your partner. I also believe that you can enjoy great foods and drink great wines without becoming obese or an alcoholic. Have you heard of the so-called French paradox? The French are renowned for eating fatty foods and drinking wine, and yet they are generally healthier, thinner, and in better shape than Americans are. Although our cholesterol levels are the same, the French have fewer heart attacks. There are a lot of possible explanations for this, one being that the French tend not to snack between meals and, while growing up, they exercise more. And the French are famous for their abilities as lovers as well! Could it be that they know something we don't about how pleasurable eating, drinking, and lovemaking fit into a healthy, balanced, cohesive lifestyle?

On a more serious note, there is no doubt that nutrition is critical to maintaining a healthy body and overall well-being, so it is important to make sure your nutritional needs are being met. Taking vitamins and supplements is good, but it is important to get as much of your nutrition as possible from fruits and vegetables.

Are you severely overweight? I don't mean "pleasingly plump," which is normal and not unhealthy. If you are clinically overweight, which means 20 to 40 percent or more above the ideal weight for your height, it may put a damper on a satisfying and loving sex life. That excess weight can directly impair your ability not only to move around during lovemaking, but also to feel sensations in your genitals and to have orgasms and erections. Men who are severely overweight often find that the fat layer over their pelvic area reduces their penis length by several inches, which becomes a direct cause of problems in making love.

If you need to lose weight, don't beat yourself up about it. Instead, focus on loving your body, and appreciating it and caring for it. Expect that it will take time and perseverance to lose weight, but that you can do it. Start eating healthy fruits and vegetables, watch your fat intake, and begin walking every day. If you need a more stringent diet or exercise program, please see your physician for advice. It may be the single best loving thing you do for yourself.

Drugs

Many people believe that certain drugs, legal or illegal, are aphrodisiacs. The bottom line is that there are no such things as aphrodisiacs. Sharing an occasional glass or two of wine or champagne with your partner may help the two of you loosen up and let go of the week's stresses, but I would not recommend this as a regular practice. Alcohol can do irreparable harm to lovemaking and loving relationships. Chronic excessive alcohol use can cause severe problems with erections, ejaculation, desire, and orgasm, not to mention the issues or conflict it can create in intimate relationships.

Some people report that they feel more sexual desire if they smoke marijuana or snort cocaine. Any positive sexual effects from these drugs are short-term. The long-term effects of all illegal drugs with which I am familiar is to impair your ability to make love and experience intimacy, on top of ruining your physical and mental health.

What about prescription drugs? Impaired sexual response is a side effect of many prescription drugs, including ulcer medications, high blood pressure medications, and even antihistamines. If you are concerned about your current sexual function and prescription drugs you are taking, consult your physician to discuss your options.

I am not a health nut or fitness buff, and prefer to spend my time talking about the positive aspects of lovemaking rather than the things that can inhibit it. But this is advice I must give: If you want to share a powerful loving, sexual bond with your partner, stop smoking, moderate your eating, drinking, and prescription medications, get some exercise, and don't use illegal drugs.

Now, on to the really fun stuff!

Chapter 6
Loving Your Partner

I n Chapters 3, 4, and 5 you learned about sensate focus touch, and how to touch slowly, sensuously, and without distraction. This is truly a form of self-love. Hopefully, you also discovered how sensate focus touch can deepen your sexual arousal and sexual pleasure. When shared between two people this touch can be very loving, and in this chapter you will find exercises that develop the loving aspects of touch.

There are more things to learn when you bring another person into the mix—about how your touch will be perceived by your partner and about the balance between enjoying yourself and knowing that your partner is enjoying herself or himself.

The caresses you will learn in this chapter are progressively more sexual and intimate, but do not involve intercourse. Before I describe them, though, I want to introduce an important aspect of sensate focus technique as it applies to partner exercises.

Active and Passive Roles

One of the issues that is not present when you caress yourself but comes up immediately when you caress a partner is performance pressure. This is the anxiety that we feel when we know that another person is paying attention to what we are doing. Performance pressure can cause thoughts like, "Am I doing this right?" and "Does she (or he) like this?"

Performance pressure inhibits us. It keeps us separate and distant from our partners, and prevents union and honest connection. In severe cases performance anxiety can drown out any sexual arousal we feel. By thinking about pleasing our partner—performing—we become separated from our bodies and our feelings. This can have an especially strong effect if we are older and are starting a new relationship. We may wonder if our new partner will respond the way our previous partner did, or whether we were doing things "the right way" all along.

By having you focus on the touch, and on the exact point of contact between your skin and your partner's skin, sensate focus exercises help you to get away from a performance orientation. Sensate focus exercises for couples have another antidote to performance pressure built into them: active and passive roles. During the following sensate focus exercises one of you will be active and one of you will be passive, then you will switch roles. Alternating activity like this helps you concentrate and will remove the pressure of feeling that you have to perform. It allows you to focus on your own touch when you are active and your partner's touch when you are passive. It will help you take greater pleasure in your touch and, most importantly, it will allow you to convey love to your partner. Breaking out of sexual roles and old patterns of expectation and response is one of the first steps toward developing sexual loving.

These active and passive roles also encourage an important aspect of wholeness, balance, and equality in your relationship. As a relationship progresses, each partner typically takes on different roles. This is especially true if you have been together for a number of years. These roles may be task-oriented or emotionally oriented, and often are unconscious. Do you cook while your partner does dishes? Are you dependent while your partner is the problem-solver? Is your partner the one who always initiates sex? You may have been together for so long that you don't even remember how some of these role divisions got started.

Loving sensate focus exercises give you the opportunity to get outside your usual roles; you have a chance to be both active and passive, and equally so. It can be scary to step outside your usual role. Try not to limit yourself by saying "I can't possibly be passive during an exercise," or "I'm just not comfortable being active." Branch out and explore a new role. Find new strengths and pleasures. Honor the importance—and the responsibility—of equality in a healthy and loving relationship.

Touching for Your Own Pleasure

The second key aspect of alternating roles is the idea that, in any exercise you do with your partner, when you are active you should touch in a way that feels good for *you*. This way of touching promotes mutuality: if you both touch for your own pleasure, you will both focus on the same thing (the touch) at the same time. You will be truly, immediately, sharing the experience.

Sometimes people think it is selfish to touch for your own pleasure or to passively accept a touch without responding, but it really is not. By establishing clear active and passive roles, sensate focus exercises take you away from expectations and interpretations. They free you to totally experience the touch without pressure, without a need to make it feel good for your partner or let him or her know it's feeling good for you.

It may be easier to feel that you are being loving toward your partner when you take the active role, but you should also be aware that as the passive partner your receptive attitude is very loving also. You are giving your partner the gift of allowing him or her to love you.

When you are active, in addition to focusing on sensations try to incorporate a mindset of positive, loving energy directed toward your partner. When you are passive, just relax and enjoy the caress. You don't have to respond in any way unless your partner is doing something that bothers you; in that case speak up gently but clearly.

The active and passive roles in the sensate focus exercises foster an intense emotional bond because you begin to learn direct, non-verbal communication instead of talking.

Before you do any of the sensate focus partner exercises it is a good idea to use some of the bonding exercises from Chapter 2. Appreciating sensual pleasure and finding nonsexual ways to bond and relax together are both critical aspects of sexual loving.

♀ Exercise ♂
Face Caress

The first sensate focus partner exercise is the "Face Caress." Too often we jump into sex and don't take time for tenderness and mutual appreciation. The "Face Caress" slows us down to appreciate the sexual pleasure of simply being close with our partner.

Before You Begin   To do this caress you will need a skin lotion that both you and your partner like, and a quiet, comfortable room in which to do the exercise. Choose a night when your children will not be around, turn on the answering machine, and secure your privacy for up to an hour.

The Exercise　This exercise is done fully clothed, but you might want to take off your shoes and belt so you are more comfortable. The active person sits with his or her back against a headboard, couch, or wall, with a pillow on the lap. The passive partner lies between the active partner's legs, head on the pillow, face up. It is important to have the passive partner's face within easy reach of the active partner.

In the face caress you stroke everything from the top of the head to the base of the neck.

Let's say the woman goes first. She begins by taking a small amount of lotion and warming it up in her hand. Then she caresses her partner's face and neck, keeping her touch very slow, light, and sensuous.

Using one or both hands, caress your partner's forehead, then move down to his cheeks, chin, and neck. Caress the bridge of his nose, his eyelids, the delicate area underneath his eyes, and his ears. Many people find touching or stroking another person's ears to be a very sensual experience.

Caress your partner for fifteen to twenty minutes, then switch roles.

The face caress is a very loving and tender exercise, and can create as much emotional closeness as it does sexual bonding. At some point you might want to change your position so you can look directly at your partner's face as you caress it, rather than seeing it upside-down. I think mature women in particular deeply appreciate having their faces touched, looked at, really seen. In addition to it being a loving act, there is a whole aspect of discovery to the face caress, as you encounter the layers of character and feeling—warmth, compassion, humor, forgiveness, vulnerability, courage, loyalty—waiting to be recognized and acknowledged. It may take men longer to reveal themselves under this caress, but once they do there are layers upon layers of pain, longing, vulnerability, and a desire to be loved waiting to be shared.

♀ Exercise ♂
Sensuous Back Caress

The back caress introduces several new elements. It is the first sensate focus exercise that involves parts of the body that you may already associate with sexual arousal, such as the buttocks. It is also the first sensate focus exercise that you do in the nude.

For you and your partner, nudity may not be an issue any more and you may be completely comfortable with each other. On the other hand, seeing each other nude may not be a comfortable part of your relationship yet. If it isn't, find ways to compromise that make you both comfortable. Start by dimming the lights. The active partner can wear a robe and drape a sheet or light blanket over the passive partner.

Before You Begin Prepare your bed (or some other comfortable place with plenty of room for both of you to stretch out), and make sure the room is warm. You may also want to use a large towel to lie on and some talcum powder. As always, make sure that you have quiet, and complete privacy. If you are a couple exploring or deepening a relationship but don't live together, and you are in the home of one of you who has children, the one who is the parent needs to make absolutely sure that children will not disturb you or otherwise embarrass you and your partner. If your partner feels any anxiety or discomfort with the situation, these exercises will not work well and may even backfire.

Spend about five minutes spoon breathing to relax together. Then decide which partner will be active first.

Let's say the man is active first. Your partner lies on her stomach on top of the towel. She may keep her arms at her sides or underneath her head—whatever is most comfortable. Then you lie next to her, maintaining as much body contact as possible during the exercise. If this isn't a comfortable position for you, try using pillows to prop your torso up or kneel next to your partner. Throughout the exercise both partners should remember the basic sensate focus instructions—focus, breathe, and relax.

The Exercise   The back caress includes your partner's entire back, from the neck to the feet, but not the genitals. As the active partner, begin by stroking your partner's back with one hand. You might want to sprinkle a little talcum powder on your hand to make your touch smoother.

Slowly run your palm or fingers over her shoulder blades, down her spine, around her buttocks. Touch to make it feel good for you. Explore the sensuality of your partner's back with different strokes, using all parts of your hand—fingertips, palm, knuckles. Pay attention to temperature, texture, contour, contrast, and shape. Run your fingers around the depression at the base of your partner's spine. Slide the tip of one finger slowly up your partner's backbone. Remember, this is not a massage, so you are not pressing or kneading her muscles.

Some areas on the back of the body that feel especially good to touch include the back of the neck, the spine, and the tender skin of the thighs underneath the buttocks. You may want to conclude the caress with a final loving or sensual gesture, like a soft pinch on the earlobe or running your fingers through your partner's hair. You will maximize your ability to focus on sensations if you close your eyes at some point during the caress.

Focus on sending a message of loving goodwill toward your partner without speaking any words. Remember to stroke your partner slowly. If you have trouble focusing, consciously slow your caressing by half the speed. If you begin to think about what your partner is feeling, gently bring your mind back to the exact point of contact between your skin and your partner's skin.

When I do the sensuous back caress I like to snuggle up against my partner and use my hand to reach as many parts of his back as I can. Then I change positions so that I can caress his legs and feet. I find that baby powder increases the pleasurable sensations for me since my hands tend to perspire, which makes my touch a little rough. Try for yourself whether powder or lotion enhances your sensations.

As a variation you can use your upper body to caress, in addition to your fingers and hand. Use your hair, face, or chest to caress if you can do it for your own pleasure and not worry about whether your partner enjoys it.

If you feel or see your partner's body becoming tense during this caress lightly pinch or press down on that muscle as a signal to relax. Remind her to breathe, and gently continue with the caress.

When you are the active partner, caress your partner's back, buttocks, and legs for your own pleasure. Think of your partner's body as a playground and touch anything that feels good to you. When you are the passive partner, simply enjoy yourself. Soak up your sensations like a sponge. Breathe deeply and evenly and relax your muscles. Keep your mind on the exact point of contact where your partner strokes you. Try not to move, just passively accept stimulation into your body. The only time you need to verbally communicate with your partner is if he or she does something that feels uncomfortable or bothers you. Spend about twenty minutes each in the active role. Between role changes hold each other and spoon breathe. Spend some time spooning again at the end of the exercise.

Some people straddle their partner's back and use both hands to do this caress. I find you experience much more feeling when the caress is done lying next to your partner, with lots of contact and a minimum of effort. In this position you feel very connected to each other and can focus on loving without being distracted by a pain or muscle cramp. Doing a back caress while straddling your partner is a more difficult position to hold, creates tension, and might set up the exercise as a performance situation for both partners.

If you become sexually aroused during the back caress, either as the active or passive partner, that's okay. Just enjoy the arousal and bring your mind back to the exact point of contact and those sensations you feel. Try not to be concerned with sexual arousal yet. Right now you are cultivating a loving touch so that it becomes second nature whenever you touch your partner. You are laying a foundation so that when you move on to exercises that are more sexual, you will exude this loving touch even when you are extremely aroused.

♀ Exercise ♂
Sensuous Front Caress

The sensuous front caress lavishes attention on the whole front of the body, from head to toe. It can include the genitals, but only in a casual way, which means that you don't spend any more time caress-ing the genitals than you do any other area. The front caress does not include penetrating the woman's vagina, only stroking outside it. This is a sensual exercise, not a sexual one, and it is not intended to arouse your partner. The instructions are the same as for the back caress: one of you caresses the other for twenty minutes, then you switch.

Before You Begin Make sure your bedroom is warm and quiet, free from distractions. If you feel more comfortable, dim the lights and slip into your robes. You will need a towel, talcum powder, and baby oil or another lubricant. Some people use Astroglide, KY jelly, or sweet almond oil. I tend to use oil-based products because oil warms up more rapidly on the body and lasts longer.

Begin with a few minutes of spoon breathing. Then let each partner pick a focusing caress—either a face caress or a back caress—to receive from the other for about five minutes, in order to shift gears and relax.

The Exercise To begin the front caress, the passive partner lies on his or her back in a relaxed position. Let's say it is the man this time. The active person lies next to him, maintaining as much full-body contact as possible. If you would like, rest your hand or your cheek on your partner's chest and listen to his heartbeat for a minute. Before you caress, sprinkle talcum powder on your partner's body and on your hand if you tend to perspire.

As the active partner, start slowly stroking your partner's body, beginning with his face, neck, shoulders, and arms. Then move down across his chest to his stomach and genitals, and finish with his legs and feet.

Caress in a flowing manner, as slowly and delicately as possible. Don't jump from the head to the legs but proceed down the body, stroking one area at a time. It is also important to maintain loving contact with your partner's body. You can help your partner relax by keeping your hands on him as much as possible and avoiding surprising or startling touches. You might like to snuggle up close to his side, maintaining contact with your legs or torso.

Throughout the caress, touch for your own pleasure. Use your palm, fingers, or the back of your hand or arm. Toward the end of the caress you may want to kneel and caress your partner's body with your face, hair, or chest. This can be very sensuous and pleasurable. Don't concern yourself with what your partner is thinking or feeling during the caress. Simply focus on bringing out loving energy toward your partner. If you caress too rapidly or roughly, your partner will feel pressured to respond. If you caress for your own enjoyment, focusing as much as you can, your partner will enjoy the caress too, and loving energy will pass between you.

When you are passive your only task is to relax and enjoy the caress. The only time you need to say or do anything is if something feels uncomfortable. If you feel yourself tensing, slow your breathing and let your body sink into the bed. Focus on the exact point of contact, receiving your partner's touch and receiving the energy in her touch. Close your eyes and focus intently on your partner's touch so that you can no longer tell where his or her hand ends and your body begins. Feel the heat radiating through your body from your partner's hand.

To finish the front caress, the active partner lies on top of or close to the passive partner and listens to his or her heart.

Spend about twenty minutes apiece on the front caress, and spoon breathe in between role changes and at the end of the exercise.

♀ Exercise ♂
Sensuous Genital Caress

Before You Begin   Come together in a warm, quiet room with a towel and a sensuous lubricant you both like. Wear robes or slip under a light sheet or blanket if you want. Center yourselves with spoon breathing. Then have each partner choose a focusing caress—either a short back caress or a short front caress—to bring you together and help you relax.

The Exercise   The passive partner (let's say it's the woman) lies comfortably on her back with her legs slightly spread. Her arms can rest at her sides or under her head, in a comfortable manner. If back pain is an issue, she should use a pillow under her knees or torso as needed.

As the active partner, begin by caressing the front of your partner's body with powder, as in the front caress. This time, however, spend at least half the time caressing your partner's genitals. After about ten minutes of the front caress, wipe the powder off your hand and warm up some lubricant in your palm. Then, slowly begin to caress your partner's genitals with your fingers.

Use lots of lubrication and slowly stroke your fingers over her outer vaginal lips, inner vaginal lips, perineum, and clitoris. Channel your attention into each stroke. Carefully insert your finger inside her vagina. Feel the warmth and texture of her vaginal walls and the muscles surrounding the vaginal opening. If your mind drifts, bring it back to your touch. Caress for ten to fifteen minutes.

If you have established sufficient intimacy so that your partner is comfortable with it, as part of this caress lie between your partner's legs as you caress her and learn what her genitals look like as well as feel like. Take this opportunity to observe the color and feel and thickness of her pubic hair, explore and learn every fold of skin, and what it hides. If you feel yourself becoming mechanical or bored with the caress, slow down your strokes.

When the woman is the active partner she should caress the front of the man's body for about ten minutes and then lubricate her fingers and slowly caress his penis and scrotum. Don't try to turn him on—caress so it feels as good as possible for you. Move your fingers around the shaft and head of the penis, and feel the ridge that separates them. Explore the feeling of the foreskin, and how it moves forward and back a little, but don't pull it back too hard (it hurts) or begin to masturbate him. Separate each testicle and run your fingers around them, holding them gently. Don't squeeze your partner's testicles—it can be quite painful for him—but do handle them. Focus on what you are feeling; if your mind drifts off to something else bring it back to your touch.

It doesn't matter whether your partner has an erection while you are doing the genital caress. A soft penis can feel just as good as an erect one—the sensations are not better or worse, just different. Experience exactly what the skin feels like on the different parts of your partner's genitals. If he becomes aroused and ejaculates, gently wipe him off and continue the caress. Caress for ten to fifteen minutes.

When you are the passive partner, close your eyes. As you receive the genital caress, focus, breathe, and relax. Allow yourself to enjoy all the sensations. The only time you need to say anything is if your partner does something that hurts or bothers you.

In between role changes, and again at the end of the exercise, come together in full-body spoon breathing. After the caress be sure to talk with each other about how each of you felt during the exercise.

♀ Exercise ♂
Sensuous Oral Sex

Continue to explore the genital caress with your partner often enough to be really comfortable with it. Then you will be ready to explore oral sex.

Sensuous oral sex is another variation of the genital caress, but, as you can imagine, you use your lips and tongue in place of your fingers. Before describing the exercise let me first say a few words about oral sex in general.

Oral sex is probably associated with more anxiety than any other sexual practice, including intercourse. Many people have never experienced oral sex because they find the idea unappealing. Others perform oral sex and do not enjoy it, or do it only to please their partner. Many sexual self-help books talk about oral sex as though there are secrets to doing it that will guarantee orgasm for your partner every time. This is very misleading. Being able to enjoy oral sex—both giving and receiving—depends more on how relaxed, loving, and focused you are than it does on any trick or technique.

If you hold negative attitudes toward oral sex, try to relax. As the genital caress should have shown you, there is nothing inherently gross or dirty about our genitals. If your partner has washed or showered recently, and is free from infection, you have nothing to worry about.

As a sex therapist and a believer in the importance of sensual loving, I encourage you to experience oral sex in the context of a sensate focus exercise. There are few things as delightful—and sexy—as giving or receiving a sensuous, pressure-free oral-genital caress. You may be surprised to find that when the performance pressure and the myths are removed from oral sex, you will most likely enjoy it greatly.

The Exercise for a Man   Start by doing a front caress with your partner, and then slowly focus on her genitals, stroking them with your hand. Have your partner lie down or sit leaning back with her legs spread apart so that you can comfortably place your face between her legs. If you are on a bed, she can prop her buttocks up with a pillow so that your neck does not get sore, or she can lie near the edge of the bed with her feet on the floor while you kneel on a pillow on the ground. Alternatively, you can sit in a chair while she stands in front of you, resting her hands on your shoulders for support. If you have issues with back or neck pain, be creative about positions that allow both of you to be comfortable during this caress.

As the active partner, do an oral caress with your tongue the same way you did a genital caress with your hand. Keep your lips, tongue, chin, and neck as relaxed as you can. Slowly move your tongue along your partner's inner thighs, outer vaginal lips, and inner vaginal lips. Let your tongue glide over her clitoris, and flick in and out of her vagina. You may also want to use your lips to softly kiss her.

Focus on the exact area of contact, and the sensations you feel. Explore how the different parts of your partner's genitals feel and taste on the different parts of your mouth. If your tongue, chin, or neck starts to get tired or sore, change positions or take a short break to relax.

Don't stiffen your tongue and rub it forcefully against her clitoris to please her, and don't forcefully suck at her vaginal lips. And don't use your fingers. If you insert a finger into her vagina or rub her clitoris while you lick her vagina, your partner will feel pressure to respond in a sexual way. Whether or not she is aware of this, she will remain anxious and will not be able to relax. The point of the exercise is for you to enjoy the sensations in your mouth and for your partner to be able to relax and enjoy herself—with no demands on her to show how much she likes it.

The Exercise for a Woman Have your partner sit or lie back in a comfortable position, and spend a few minutes on a front caress. Then move your caress to your partner's genitals for a few minutes until you are both focused and relaxed. Lower your head to your partner's pelvis and slowly use your tongue and lips to lick all over his inner thighs and penis and scrotum. Explore freely, and do what makes your tongue feel good. You can lick the area behind his testicles, and trace your tongue along the creases between his thighs and scrotum. You may want to take his whole penis into your mouth and slowly let it back out again. Experience how each different area feels and tastes on your lips and tongue.

You can do this caress regardless of whether your partner has an erection or not. Don't put pressure on your partner or yourself. Think of your own pleasure, not your partner's. Keep your tongue and lips relaxed, not stiff. Don't suck on his penis in such a way that your head moves up and down. If your neck or tongue becomes tired or sore, move into a different position or take a short break. If you feel pressured to perform, stop and caress some other part of your partner's body until you feel that you are focused enough to enjoy the oral caress again. Respond to what you want, and put what your partner wants out of your mind.

If your partner indicates that he is about to ejaculate, you can decide whether to take the semen in your mouth or whether to stop the caress while your partner ejaculates. If you are not through with the caress, wipe off the semen and continue. There is a possibility that this might be a sensitive issue for one or both of you, with implications of acceptance or lack of it. In that case it is best to discuss the question beforehand and resolve what you will do, so that there isn't tension during the exercise when the possibility of ejaculation arises.

Use only your mouth for this caress. Don't use your hand to masturbate your partner. Remember that you are doing this caress only for your own pleasure and to convey love to your partner. It doesn't matter whether your partner gets aroused, has an erection, or ejaculates. What does matter is that you do what feels good for you and that you focus on the sensations in your mouth during the caress.

Peaking and Plateauing with a Partner

How did you like those caresses? Did you enjoy spending quiet, sensual time together without sex as the spoken or unspoken goal? Did you feel something shift in the way you experienced touching each other as you took on the active and passive roles? Over time these subtle shifts can make profound changes in the quality of your relationship.

The following exercises introduce you to exploring your arousal levels with a partner. In Chapter 5, you learned to peak at high arousal levels by yourself. Peaking and prolonged states of arousal are a vital part of making love better than ever because this wave-like arousal pattern brings about optimal, continued release of endorphins and intensifies orgasm. As you share the intimate process of peaking and plateauing with your lover, you may find it a dynamic, passionate experience both physically and emotionally.

♀ Exercise ♂
Peaking with Your Partner

The Exercise Let's begin with the woman active and the man passive. The man lies on his back while the woman begins with a front caress and then moves to a genital caress. As his arousal climbs, the man tells his partner the level he has reached. For example, when his arousal reaches a "strong" level he tells his partner so. She stops the caress and allows his arousal to decrease to a more gentle level. When the man calls out that his arousal level is "gentle," the woman begins caressing him again. The couple repeats this rising, peaking, and subsiding arousal pattern, with each peak getting a little higher, until the man peaks into orgasm.

This is just like peaking by yourself only now you are completely passive, savoring your partner's touch and communicating your arousal to her or him. You can do this exercise using a manual caress or an oral caress for as long as you like, then switch roles.

You can learn a lot about the subtleties of your partner's arousal cycle by paying close attention to the changes in his or her breathing and heartbeat. Does he radiate heat when aroused? Does her face and chest flush when her arousal heightens? When you end your role as the active partner, lightly place your hand or face on your partner's heart and listen, or cuddle up next to your partner and spoon breathe.

♀ Exercise ♂
Plateauing with Your Partner

Remember that plateauing is very similar to peaking, but here the focus is on maintaining a certain level of arousal. As we said in Chapter 5, there are four ways to plateau: by changing your breathing, changing your focus, using your PC muscle, and changing your movements.

Begin with some kissing or cuddling and a short focusing caress. Have one partner be passive first, then switch roles.

The Exercise   This time let's have the man be active first. His partner lies on her back while he does a front and genital caress to stir her arousal. Then he continues sensuous genital caresses with his hands or mouth, as he desires.

As the passive partner you accept your partner's delicate touch, letting your arousal build to a "strong" level. Then, while your partner continues his caresses, you try to hover at that strong level for a few moments and not go higher by slowing and deepening your breathing. If you slip below this strong level, speed up your breathing to increase your arousal.

Hovering like this takes intense concentration on both your own responses and the stimulation your partner provides for you. It really helps that you don't have to feel responsible for how your partner is doing, and whether or not he is enjoying himself.

For the next plateau, try to maintain your arousal level by doing pelvic rolls or thrusts while your partner continues to caress your genitals. Begin with sensuous pelvic movements when you feel somewhat aroused, then speed up the movements until you reach a very strong level. If you feel your arousal heading toward "urgent," slow your thrusting down a bit so you can hover at the very strong level. After a while speed up the rolls and thrusts to allow your arousal to climb to urgent again.

For the third plateau use your PC muscle to take your arousal down and pelvic rolls and thrusts to bring it back up. See if you can begin to recognize more subtle changes in your arousal level.

For the last plateau try switching your focus from one part of your body to another, and try to plateau at an "urgent" level. As you go into urgent arousal, mentally switch your focus from the part of your genitals that your partner is caressing to some other part. This will lower your arousal level slightly. Then switch your focus back to the area being touched in order to climb to urgent and beyond.

If you feel like having an orgasm after the last plateau let yourself fall into one, but don't feel like you have to.

With practice you will soon be able to use all the techniques at each plateau without having to think about them, and you and your partner should be able to maintain your arousal level within a narrow range that you are able to control. You will be able to recognize quite subtle changes in your arousal level, such as the different gradations between somewhat strong, strong, very strong, almost urgent, and so forth.

Now that you have tapped into basic sexual loving with caresses of the face, the back, the front, and the genitals, you are ready to explore the more advanced loving exercises in the next few chapters. As you develop your repertoire, keep in mind that you can always come back to these exercises. Front and back caresses are wonderful ways to cherish and honor each other's bodies, and can also be used as foreplay for longer lovemaking sessions.

Chapter 7

Loving Intercourse

Now is the time to come together in the ultimate loving connection—intercourse. The word "intercourse" means communication, and making love can be all that and more. This chapter offers you many ways to have intercourse while exploring different loving mindsets.

Although what follows contains short descriptions of different ways to have intercourse, these aren't different positions or "recipes" for sex, as you would find in a typical sex manual. Rather, they are intimate ways of relating physically and expressing love. The suggestions I make are simply that, suggestions. They are based on my experience and the positions are ones that seem to best convey love and increase sexual pleasure. Use them as jumping off points for the ways in which you want to and are inspired to come together.

If you are a couple in a relatively new relationship, you may have already had intercourse before you made a joint decision to try this program of sexual loving. Even so this can be a significant threshold for both of you. It is very important, before you try any of these exercises, to be sure that you are ready for them. You need to feel trust in each other and openness to the experience. If you feel pressured or harbor a current resentment toward your partner, it will prevent you from being able to fully let go and connect with him or her. And if you are not comfortable with the idea of expressing self-love for your body, you will also feel inhibited. In that case talk it over with your partner and go back and do some of the earlier exercises, either together or alone.

When you have intercourse, use whichever positions are comfortable for the two of you. If you have back, knee, or any other physical problems, talk about them with your partner in advance. At this level of a relationship it is far better to be open and honest than to try and conceal issues that may have a negative impact on your health or physical well-being. Be creative and considerate of each other; use pillows or cushions to ensure your comfort; ensure that your time together is undisturbed and private; jointly create an atmosphere that is conducive to affection and arousal.

The time before intercourse is very important. You need it to get centered and in sync with each other, and to relax and focus on your arousal. It is very important to spend time spoon breathing, and to spend time holding and caressing each other in nonsexual and sexual ways. You may also wish to spend time with oral caresses and sensuous oral sex. After intercourse, maintain physical contact and take time to spoon breathe together or nurture each other in an embrace.

You will need a "coming down" period to re-ground yourselves after the experience of loving intercourse.

If you decide to have intercourse after doing another, non-intercourse exercise, remember your basics. Relax and open to your loving mindset. Allow yourselves time so you don't feel rushed. And get centered together by beginning with spoon breathing and a focusing caress.

♀ Exercise ♂
Goal-Free Intercourse

The idea behind goal-free intercourse is to escape the pressure to have—and to give—an orgasm. Intercourse without orgasm nurtures an understanding of the continuity between skin sensuality, foreplay, and intercourse. As you enjoy goal-free intercourse you learn to be more flexible and indulgent in your lovemaking. You learn to not think of intercourse as the *result* of foreplay, or of orgasm as the necessary end result of intercourse. Surprisingly, many couples discover that learning this goal-free orientation leads them to stronger orgasms.

The Exercise   First decide who will be active and who will be passive. If the woman is active, she begins by doing a sensate focus caress with her partner—front, genital, and oral. When he gets an erection, she climbs onto him and begins thrusting with slow, sensuous strokes for as long as she desires. Her partner remains passive and doesn't move; his responsibility is to focus on the pleasurable sensations he feels and receive his partner's movements.

There should be no performance pressure, no goals, no thinking ahead, and no orgasm. After a short while the woman maintains the sexual connection by lowering herself into an embrace with her partner.

When the man is active, the woman lies on her back or reclines on supportive pillows. Her only responsibility is to focus on her own sensations. Her partner does a front caress, and genital and oral caresses until she is relaxed enough for him to enter her. If he likes, he can kneel and use his penis to caress her labia and the outside of her vagina. When he is ready for intercourse, he can put a pillow underneath his partner, raise her legs, and enter her. This position, in which the woman raises her legs and the man kneels between them, brings you into a lovely face-to-face connection and offers greater stimulation for both. (If you have trouble kneeling you can also use the missionary position.)

The man makes slow, sensuous strokes, as he desires, and when finished lies lovingly on top of or beside his partner.

♀ Exercise ♂
Sensate Focus Intercourse

This is intercourse with a different focus—sensuality. In previous chapters you practiced focusing on skin sensations in all parts of the body. With sensate focus intercourse you focus on the erotic sensations of the penis in the vagina.

The Exercise with the Man Active Ask your partner to lie comfortably on her back, and do sensuous caresses, including a front caress, a genital caress, or an oral-genital caress. If you need direct stimulation to have an erection, use your penis to caress your partner's vagina, or caress yourself with your hand.

When you are ready, start intercourse in the kneeling position described in the exercise above. As the active partner, you control the speed of thrusting. Thrust as slowly as possible, trying to caress all parts of your partner's vagina with your penis. Both of you should feel free to move, to thrust and roll with each other while focusing on the exquisite sensations of your penis inside her vagina.

Next, try switching your focus from how your penis feels to how her vagina feels around your penis. After a while try to switch focus to different parts of your penis. What do you feel—warmth, slickness, tantalizing friction? Both of you should focus on the same sensations at the same time. Gaze at each other as you focus and direct your loving intentions through the dual connection of your genitals and your eyes.

There should be no pressure from either of you to have an orgasm, but if you do that is okay. As the active partner, you decide when intercourse is over; bring your movements to a slow and sensuous rest, and embrace your partner.

The Exercise with the Woman Active Ask your partner to lie on his back as you do a front caress, a genital caress, and perhaps oral sex. When he has an erection, climb on top and begin slowly thrusting on his penis. Think of it as caressing his penis with your vagina. Both of you should focus on the sensations of his penis inside your vagina.

As the active partner, you lead in the speed and extent of thrusting, and your partner follows. It's like dancing—in fact it *is* a dance, a love dance. As you make love, look into each other's eyes and try to match your breathing. It is not important if either or both of you has an orgasm. Since you are the active partner, the exercise is over whenever you decide to stop. Slow your movements down and lower yourself into an embrace.

♀ Exercise ♂
Loving Intercourse

Loving intercourse is also intercourse freed from pressure and goals. It is intercourse that focuses on tapping into the sexual energy and loving connection the two of you share. In loving intercourse you visualize and project your loving sexual energy toward your partner, combining your attention with your intention.

The Exercise with the Woman Active Caress your partner while you both center your energies together. Focus on bringing your mind and emotions fully into the present. Then, focus that energy on each other.

When your partner has a partial or full erection, climb on top and begin intercourse. While thrusting and focusing, visualize your vagina as a vessel that surrounds your partner's penis. Imagine that your vagina is filled with warmth and energy, giving out a white, loving light that flows into your partner.

This visualization will convey a positive loving energy from your vagina to your partner's penis. If your partner focuses on the same visualization you will find your vagina actually feels hot during intercourse.

There is no goal, no pressure, and no time limit. You decide when the exercise is over. If you are able to reach a climax, give your partner the ultimate loving energy gift of your very intense orgasm.

The Exercise with the Man Active Caress your partner while you both center your energies together. Gently caress her genitals, perhaps with sensuous oral sex. Both of you should focus on bringing your mind and emotions fully into the present. When your partner is aroused and lubricated, begin intercourse in the kneeling position (or another position that works for you).

Visualize your penis as a loving instrument, radiating loving energy to your partner. Or think of your sexual energy as a blue or white light flowing into your partner. If both of you focus on the visualization, you will feel the heat of this energy in your penis. You can continue with intercourse as long as you want to, with or without an orgasm.

Sometimes it is easier for a man to do this visualization because, if he has an orgasm, he actually is pouring something into his partner. For women it is important to realize that your orgasm can be a real energy gift—powerful, hot, and loving.

♀ Exercise ♂
Heart Awareness Intercourse

During heart awareness intercourse you listen to your lover's heartbeat as the rhythms of your lovemaking build and climax. This form of intercourse creates an incredible bonding experience, especially if one or both of you has an orgasm. It's certainly not something to be undertaken by the faint of heart, so to speak. Heart awareness intercourse sharpens your knowledge of the rhythms of your bodies, of your arousal, and ultimately, of each other. It makes you acutely aware of the fragile, persistent, very human nature of your partner—and it shows you how strongly your partner is affected by your presence.

If the position of listening to your partner's heart isn't comfortable for you, adjust your position so that your hearts are against each other and beat together as you make love.

The Exercise with the Woman Active   Relax and hold each other, then spend time caressing each other and becoming aware of your arousal. When you are ready, straddle your partner and begin thrusting sensuously.

While making love, lean over and rest your ear on your partner's chest. Feel his warmth. Listen to your heartbeat as you both become more and more aroused. See if you can cause his heartbeat to speed up or slow down with the speed and force of your thrusting. As his heart beats faster does his breathing quicken? Does your arousal climb? Does *your* heart beat faster?

The Exercise with the Man Active   Relax and hold each other, then spend time caressing each other and becoming aware of your arousal. When you are ready, kneel between your partner's legs and enter her slowly. As you thrust into her sensuously, lean over so your ear rests on your partner's chest. Feel her warmth and listen to her heartbeat. Does the speed and passion of your thrusting affect the beating of her heart? Does her breathing quicken? Does your arousal climb in tandem?

If you feel like it, continue making love while you maintain some connection with your hearts. If one or both of you orgasms, focus on the energy that pours out of your heart as you climax. Let the energy flow through your bodies, and listen to or feel each other's heartbeat gradually slow down. Hold each other close and breathe together until your hearts both beat at a resting pace.

Now here are some intercourse exercises intended to deepen and enrich your arousal. They teach you to peak and plateau during intercourse, while you take turns being active. Realizing the potential of your arousal unleashes your full sexual energy, and fosters a strong sense of mutuality. I hope you will find new pleasure and passion with these.

♀ Exercise ♂
Peaking Together

There are several ways to peak together, depending on which of you is active and who is on top. I will describe four options. If these inspire you to create new positions, go for it. Keep in mind that it doesn't matter how highly aroused you become in any exercise. With mutual agreement you can always stop the exercise and have regular intercourse or exchange loving caresses. Orgasm is not the goal, though it will be delicious if you go there.

The time frame on all these peaking exercises is about twenty minutes to half an hour, give or take a few minutes. During a twenty-minute exercise most people are comfortable doing about five peaks and taking four or five minutes for the up and down phases of the peak. Depending on your personal response style you can compress the peaks or lengthen them. Do what feels comfortable and pleasing.

During the peaking exercises, both of you should feel or visualize the peaks as waves. At first you may not peak together, but with time you will become so in tune with each other's bodies and arousal that your arousal will develop mutually and build upon each other's. Together you may reach new heights.

Before beginning intercourse, make sure you have spent plenty of time kissing and caressing each other, and are aroused and ready for intercourse.

Man on Top, Man Peaking   Start intercourse in a kneeling position. Let your partner know when you begin to reach a strong level of arousal. Then stop, or slow down. Do this not to keep from ejaculating but to create the energy-wave pattern that releases endorphins. Try peaking at increasingly stronger levels of arousal. If your partner is able to follow the peaks with you, that's great. With practice she will learn to read your body and intuit your arousal, so there will be no need to say your arousal level out loud. If you have an orgasm during this exercise, I guarantee it will be explosive.

Man on Top, Woman Peaking　Start intercourse in a kneeling position, but this time your partner gives you the feedback. When she tells you she has reached a strong level of arousal, then you slow down. She can signal you to start thrusting again with a touch on your chest. Bring her to a few more peaks at increasingly strong and then urgent levels. Can you follow her up to the point where you orgasm together? With practice you will be able to do so.

Woman on Top, Woman Peaking　Start intercourse astride your partner. Thrust sensuously on your partner until you reach a strong level of arousal, then let your partner know. Slow down your movements to peak, then speed them up again to increase your arousal. Control all your own peaks through the strong and urgent levels of arousal until you climax or feel that you are satiated. If you do reach orgasm, I'll bet the intensity or how long it lasts will surprise you.

Woman on Top, Man Peaking　Start intercourse astride your partner and respond to him as he gives you feedback about his arousal level. When he reaches a strong arousal level, stop and start or slow your movements to let him peak. He can speak or lightly touch your back to let you know when to begin thrusting again. Bring him to peaks at stronger and then urgent levels of arousal, until he reaches the edge of climax. Then move with the explosiveness of his orgasm. If you keep your movements sensuous and slow, both of you will feel every loving stroke.

After you feel satiated—which may be after one or both of you have had orgasms or not, or just when you feel satisfied—settle into a loving embrace. Kiss or stroke your partner, or gaze into each other's eyes. After the release of sexual energy in this exercise it is important to keep a connection between the two of you.

♀ Exercise ♂
Plateauing with Intercourse

Plateauing with intercourse is a more challenging adventure. Remember that when you plateau, you coast at a particular arousal level for a few seconds up to a few minutes. Plateauing, especially at very high arousal levels, can give you a maximum endorphin release and create an altered state of consciousness. At these high levels of arousal you may experience a wonderful distortion of time, so that even the plateaus that last a few seconds seem to last a lot longer.

Remember also that there are four techniques you can use to maintain a plateau: the PC muscle squeeze, deep breathing, pelvic movements, and shifting focus. The one you make the most use of in the following exercises is breathing.

Again, before heading into intercourse you and your partner should take time breathing together, cuddling, and caressing each other. To feel comfortable with these high levels of arousal you need to feel grounded in each other and focused on your bodies' pleasure.

Man on Top, Man Plateauing Start intercourse in a kneeling position, and begin to move sensuously in your partner. Bring your arousal to a peak as you head into a strong level of arousal. Then let it plateau a few times at stronger levels. When it hits each plateau and starts to climb a little, slow down your movements and breathing and slip back to a lesser level of strong arousal.

Then speed up your breathing, and climb to an urgent level of arousal. Hover there for several seconds, and plateau using your breath as you need to. At this stage your breathing will almost be panting, your sensations will be very intense, and you will feel as if you are almost hyperventilating to stay on the edge.

At the moment of orgasm, open your eyes wide and take a deep breath.

Man on Top, Woman Plateauing Arouse your partner with manual and oral caresses until she is ready for intercourse. After you start intercourse, your partner will let you know as she peaks at strong and stronger levels of arousal. Based on her feedback, slow down or speed up your movements. She will control her plateaus at stronger and urgent levels of arousal by alternately slowing her breathing and panting. She can also hover at certain plateaus by changing her pelvic movements or squeezing her PC muscle.

Woman on Top, Woman Plateauing Arouse your partner with manual and oral caresses until he is erect and ready for intercourse. Then climb astride your partner and use his penis to pleasure yourself. Sensuously stroke yourself and thrust up and down to build your arousal. Peak and plateau at increasingly stronger levels of arousal by controlling the speed of your movements and your breathing. See if you can hover at these plateaus up to a minute. If you fall into orgasm, open your eyes wide and take a deep breath.

Woman on Top, Man Plateauing Make sure your partner is aroused and erect, and ready for intercourse. During intercourse you will thrust and move on your partner, slowing down as he gives you feedback for his lower level peaks. Your partner will control his plateaus at stronger and urgent levels of arousal by alternately slowing his breathing and panting. He can also hover at certain plateaus by changing his pelvic movements or squeezing his PC muscle.

When intercourse has concluded, you and your partner may feel both exhausted and energized. You may find that your minds are clearer and your senses sharpened, while your bodies are fully relaxed. Take advantage of this to enjoy each other and share the pleasures you have just experienced.

♀ Exercise ♂
Mutuality Intercourse

For this exercise you can have intercourse in whatever position feels comfortable or inspires you at the time. The idea is to try to see and feel the intercourse from the viewpoint of your partner. In doing so you will find that you cannot tell where you end and your partner begins. You will feel ultimately unified, a greater whole than each of you individually.

The Exercise   There are a few different ways to experience mutual intercourse. The first is to begin with peaking, so you are at higher arousal levels when you start intercourse. As the man penetrates, ask yourself, "Is what I feel the penis or the vagina?" If you are a woman, see if you can put your consciousness in your partner's penis. If you are a man, see if you can put your consciousness in your partner's vagina.

The second way to experience mutuality is to enjoy your usual lovemaking style, but as you get into it pretend your positions are reversed. If you are on top, close your eyes and imagine you are on the bottom. If you are on the bottom, close your eyes and visualize yourself on top. As you both mutually concentrate on this visualization and continue making love you will feel a sensation that the two of you are spinning or whirling together through space.

A third way to experience mutuality is to begin your lovemaking in your usual style but to try to place your consciousness in the body of your partner. As you thrust and move, focus on what the movement and the intercourse feel like from your partner's perspective. Try to visualize that you are your partner, moving against yourself. As your partner does the same you may experience a deep sense of unity and mutuality.

• • •

The styles of intercourse in this chapter are sensual and fun, and they can also be profoundly moving. You can use them as exercises to focus on each other and your sexual connection, and include them regularly into your lovemaking to deepen your pleasure. Keep in mind that they can only really help you make your love better when both of you come together willingly and expressively, ready to give yourselves over—jointly—to deep arousal and intense sexual pleasure. Before and after intercourse always spend the time you need treasuring each other and each other's body.

Chapter 8
Loving to Play

A lot of our unstructured lovemaking serves the same function for us as adults that play does for children. It lets us relax and take the pressure off ourselves. It is dynamic, creative, expressive, and unself-conscious. Unlike most activities in our adult lives, lovemaking isn't goal-oriented—or at least it shouldn't be. And it is true that the family that plays together stays together. If you and your partner wish to enrich your relationship, one of the greatest things you can do together is play, whether it is sports or any other games you both enjoy.

The capacity to play is very important to our overall enjoyment of life, to keeping us in touch with the creative, child-like, funny, and romantic parts of ourselves. A grown person's willingness to play is often a good indicator of a capacity to be open to exploring new ways of sexual loving and fulfillment. If I were starting a new relationship after forty I would make a healthy playfulness—one that was not overly focused on competitiveness or one-sided teasing—one of the key qualities that I would look for in a new partner. If I was rebuilding or deepening a relationship with a long-term partner I would want him or her to commit to playing with me in new and more mutual ways every day.

If you have always seen yourself as "serious" or somewhat inhibited, don't worry. It is seldom hard to get back in touch with the playful child in each of us, though it may take a little time. Start by increasing the time you spend on play activities you currently enjoy. These can range from indoor games like doing crosswords (start doing them with your partner, maybe invent a game of "strip crosswords"), playing cards (strip poker), and silent charades (strip charades?) to outdoor sports and activities where it may be best to keep your clothes on! Keep your games light and enjoyable, and not too competitive unless you can both handle competition without becoming sore losers. The idea is to focus on how both of you win new intimacy by playing together, not how one of you can win by defeating the other or sulking because you don't like the game.

You can also add in silliness, which is an important part of play. Again, this may range from tickling to singing nonsense verse you sang as a kid to recalling silly jokes to dressing in absurd ways. Try it all—especially those things you remember doing as a kid that everyone would call "weird." Remember, in private the weird can be wonderful. And when your partner is weird back at you, take time to appreciate and enjoy it, and join in if you can without taking over.

As your willingness to play together and the time you spend playing increases, add in some of the romantically playful exercises below.

For most of them I have given fairly basic guidelines for you to explore, embroider, improvise around, change, take to ridiculous extremes, whatever. One of the key aspects of successful, trusting play is not getting too hung up on the rules of the game. But *do* respect the rules of engagement: physically hurting each other is not okay; everyone gets time to be "it," whatever it is; remember you're playing together to get closer and share good loving; and the idea is to have fun!

♀ Exercise ♂
Sensuous Bath or Shower

The sensuous bath or shower is a whole-body caress that takes place in the bathtub or shower. The purpose of the sensuous bath is not to get clean (though you probably will), but to enjoy your own body and your partner's body in a different way, with added sensations.

There are a number of ways to savor a sensuous bath. You can sexily soap and caress each other's face and body. You can romantically bathe the other person, and wash and comb each other's hair. You can be silly and give each other colorful facials. Or you can heat up the water with sensuous oral sex. You can alternate taking active and passive roles, or you can mutually caress each other at the same time. And don't forget that you can caress with all the different parts of your body, not just your fingers.

Try using a fragrant bath gel or foaming bath oil, and caress any parts of your partner's body that feel good. Touch with all parts of your body. When you caress, touch for your own pleasure. Focus on the silky sensations of your partner's wet skin and hair. When you receive a caress, concentrate on exactly where you are being touched, just as you would during any sensate focus exercise.

If you become aroused during the caress simply allow yourself to experience the arousal. Don't try to heighten your arousal or push it away, just relax into it. Enjoy the feelings of your partner caressing you and the water beating down on your skin. It you feel inspired to carry your play over into intercourse, go for it. But remember that intercourse shouldn't be the goal of the sensuous shower or bath—the only goal here is good, clean fun!

After your bath don't forget to pat each other dry with warm towels and a loving touch.

♀ Exercise ♂
Tom Jones Dinner

Many of us gobble our food or eat while doing other things. We fail to take the time to enjoy the simple, sensuous aspects of eating. Now here is your opportunity!

The Tom Jones Dinner is named after the incredibly indulgent eating scene in the movie of the same name. When I was in surrogate training, we did this exercise as part of our training. Everyone in the class (ten to twelve people) brought some type of sweet or savory food that could be eaten with the hands. We spread a sheet out on the floor and laid out the foods beautifully. We were all nude—this was the Seventies, after all—and there were three rules: no feeding yourself, no talking, and no using utensils. Everybody fed each other. Some of these dinners got pretty wild, but the point of the dinner was not to have a wild food orgy. It was to learn to enjoy the purely sensuous aspects of eating, free from the restraints of table manners.

You can create a Tom Jones Dinner at home for you and your partner. First, choose some sensuous foods. Things that are creamy or juicy will feel especially good in your mouth. Think of slick, slippery, sweet, savory, and sticky foods. You might consider fruits, especially juicy ones such as oranges and peaches, hors d'oeuvres such as cheese and crackers, any juicy meat that can be pulled off the bone, and anything messy that can be licked off fingers and body parts. For beverages serve wine or champagne, sparkling water, or fruit juice. For dessert try strawberries and whipped cream or a chocolate mousse.

Arrange the food on a sheet to protect your carpeting and furniture. Take off your clothes or undress each other. Pour each other a drink, make a toast, and then begin to feed each other. Go slowly, and savor both the food and your partner feeding it to you. Eat with the goal of feeling every sensation as the food passes your lips and through your mouth. Watch your partner eat. Place food on your partner's body and slowly lick it off, or offer food to your partner on yours. If you want a drink, take a drink and then, with a kiss, share it with your partner.

Finish the Tom Jones Dinner by washing each other off with warm, wet towels or taking a sensuous shower.

♀ Exercise ♂
Role-Playing

We have all heard of couples who occasionally dress up or role-play "Pirate and Wench" or "Hooker and Client." A lot of couples have found that different forms of role-playing are harmless and intriguing, and really get them excited. I don't like to make specific suggestions for couples, because role-playing depends on the context of your relationship and the ways in which you like to experiment. Your preferred role-playing could be an interpersonal change that alters the usual sexual roles you choose in the relationship, or it can be more of a fantasy enactment. For example, for some couples having the partner who usually instigates sex and leads in lovemaking be passive (or vice versa) is a daring, satisfying experience. Other couples might experiment with playing out characters in a dramatic encounter. Some couples like to take the role-play outside their bedroom, or even outside the house.

The type of role-playing I suggest for beginners lies somewhere in the middle. If you are a woman, pretend that you are highly arousable and highly orgasmic and carry this all the way through a session of lovemaking. If you are a man, pretend that you are a stereotyped version of a great lover and carry this all the way through a session of lovemaking. Another way to do this is to pretend you are the opposite sex. If you are a woman, pretend that you are a man while making love. If you are a man, pretend that you are a woman. This can get quite intense if you get in touch with basic gender identity aspects of your personality and their role in the dynamics of your relationship.

Role-playing, besides being fun, can help you see sides of yourself that you didn't know existed. A lot of people find that fantasy adds to their arousal during lovemaking, but they often feel guilty about doing it, or feel they are being unfaithful to their partner. But acting as if you are another person or as if you are making love to a person other than your partner can actually be a growth experience. If you share this with each other beforehand, it can increase your intimacy. And the sexual fun you can have discovering your partner's different, perhaps hidden sexual expressions can bring you both closer in ways you never foresaw, or could imagine.

If you and your partner are more theatrical, try exploring new roles. Some of these sexual role-plays may be a bit of a stretch at first, but here are some scenarios to get you started:

- Pirate and Serving Wench
- Rock Star and Groupie (male and female, or same sex!)
- Nurse and Patient
- Slave and Master or Mistress
- Farmer's Daughter and Traveling Salesman
- Cowboy and Barmaid
- Housewife and Delivery Boy
- Sex Guru and Disciple
- Damsel and Knight in Shining Armor
- Pervert and Innocent
- High School Sweethearts
- Cheerleader and Stud
- Homecoming Queen (King) and Class Geek . . . .

♀ Exercise ♂
Body Decoration

How often have you heard it said that the body is sacred? And how long has it been since you worshipped your lover's body? Here is a simple way to start. Buy some body paints that are suitable for use on the skin. You should be able to find these at a bath shop, an adult store, or through a catalog. You could also use a henna kit that is used to create temporary mehndi tattoos. Or, if you're feeling silly, pick up some children's bath paints in rainbow or pastel colors.

Set aside some creative time and sequester yourselves in your bathroom or a secluded, private area outside if you have one. Undress each other and offer each other your body as a canvas. Take turns painting each other's body. You may wish to paint symbols that mean something to both of you, or designs that celebrate your body and body parts. In keeping with the theme of this chapter, you can cover your partner's body with playful designs. Use brushes or sponges to paint with or use your fingers. And when you are both painted, do whatever you are inspired to do! If the paints are edible, lick them off. (If you're really indulgent, you can have a Tom Jones dinner and cover yourselves with food as well as paint!) Then take a sensuous shower together to wash the paint off.

♀ Exercise ♂
Mutual Masturbation

Masturbation is one of the most personal, intimate things that we experience. Many of us feel it is so private that we are hesitant to share this experience with a partner. One of the best ways to begin to share is to do it in the spirit of play. It may help to picture yourself masturbating the first time you did it, or picture yourself as a child when you touched yourself. Try to remember how good it felt, and what it was like to be that excitable, before self-consciousness and shyness set in.

There are a few ways to share mutual masturbation. One is for both of you to masturbate at the same time. You can undress in front of the other person, then lie together on the bed, without touching, and stimulate yourself the way you would if you were alone. Pay attention to your own arousal and send that energy out to your partner. If you wish, look at each other as you become more and more aroused. If you get the urge to giggle or even laugh, do it! That's what this exercise is all about.

Another way to do this is to take turns masturbating while the other watches. Again, you can undress in front of each other, then lie back and get comfortable. Relax your body and inhibitions. Close your eyes and pleasure yourself the way you like to most. The more you can let go the more pleasurable this will be for both you and your partner.

♀ Exercise ♂
Delicate Restraint

If you and your partner are feeling a bit adventurous, and you feel really comfortable with your trust in each other, you might enjoy breaking out some delicate bondage. Silk stockings, neckties, scarves, and similar pieces of clothing—with a little bit of creativity and passion—can be transformed into the most luxurious restraints. This playful enterprise puts a new spin on passive and active roles. I promise you, you won't look at that necktie the same way again!

When you are active, seductively restrain your partner. You can use your bedposts, or simply tie his or her wrists together. (If this is his or her first time, do so gently and loosely.) Then use your partner's body to pleasure yourself. Be playful, lustful, expressive, indulgent. After you have had your way, kiss your partner warmly, let your partner go, and roll over. It's your partner's turn next!

When you are passive, relax as much as you can and relish all the sensations. Tell your partner if anything feels uncomfortable or painful. Nothing about this play should be painful or degrading.

Many people are aroused by being tied up because it feels kinky and a little bit dangerous. You will find that doing this together increases your intimacy, and emphasizes the degree to which you can trust each other.

If you and your partner have tried or enjoyed restraints before and are interested in different textures, most adult catalogs and adult boutiques carry fur-lined cuffs, Velcro cuffs, leather restraints, and more.

♀ Exercise ♂
Naked Sundays

This is a cross between a game and a couple ritual, and probably works best if you are at an age where your children don't live at home any more and are unlikely to visit. (It could also be another reason not to let them move back in with you!)

As the name suggests, once you have brought in the Sunday paper, make all your time indoors for the rest of the day clothing optional. If you have a sequestered back yard or live far enough away from others, you can take this out of doors as well. You don't have to do anything special, but over time this will begin to feel like an essential freedom and can give you a new sense of intimacy and appreciation of the natural, unguarded beauty of the human body. And loving intercourse, using one of the suggestions in this book, can be a great way to fill that lazy Sunday afternoon.

Keep robes by the door in case someone comes calling. And don't forget to wear an apron if you're frying bacon or flipping pancakes for brunch!

♀ Exercise ♂
The Nature Connection

Remember that old movie *Splendor in the Grass*? The title comes from a poem by William Wordsworth that I really like, "Ode on Intimations of Immortality From Recollections of Early Childhood." The exact quote is "Though nothing can bring back the hour of splendor in the grass, of glory in the flower."

What does this have to do with making love better than ever? The poem is about how we perceive things differently when we are kids—how we would take the time to study a blade of grass, or an insect, and wonder at the mystery and beauty of it. So many of us spend our days staring out at the very unsexy landscape of buildings, cars, smog, computers, you name it. Nature is sexy.

Your ability to recapture that youthful sense of innocence and wonder is essential to rejuvenating your love life. And believe it or not, that is something that begins outside of the bedroom. I find that the best way to start is to venture outdoors. I'm sure you can find some area of natural beauty near your own home. It doesn't matter whether it's the desert, the beach, the mountains, or the forest—even contemplation of the night sky will do. Just make sure you take time to wander and wonder, and share it with your partner.

Escape with your partner to a location you both agree on. Take some food, take a little wine if you drink alcohol, and have a picnic. Read each other some poetry. After you eat, maybe you can make out a little and perhaps fall asleep. If you are in a private location and feel amorous, go for it!

Chapter 9
Loving Desire

A s a sex therapist who has written several self-help books, I appear frequently on television to discuss sexual issues. In many cases the host opens up the show to questions from a studio audience or people calling in from home. The question I am most frequently asked is some version of, "How do I put the spark, the passion, back in my love life?" What these people are really asking about is how to increase their sexual desire.

Sex Drive versus Sexual Desire

Sexual desire is a topic that is confusing even to sex therapists. The 1980s saw a tremendous increase in what sex therapists call "hypo-active sexual desire disorder" or low sex drive. Interestingly enough, there is no corresponding disorder to describe someone who has an abnormally high sex drive. What actually happened in the 1980s is that sex therapists gave diagnostic labels to people's behavior, despite not knowing or having an understanding of what "sexual desire" is.

Sex therapists have described sexual desire as the feeling that you want sex or the tendency to fantasize about sex. But we do not have any objective measure of sexual desire. We only have measures of how frequently a couple makes love, and frequency does not equal desire. I believe we can clear up some of the confusion here by distin-guishing between "sexual desire" and "sex drive."

Sex drive is fired by the hormone testosterone in both men and women. (Contrary to most people's impression, although testosterone is a male hormone, women produce testosterone too, but in much smaller amounts.) Sexual desire, on the other hand, is a complex interaction in which our mood, self-consciousness, intimate relation-ship, and external circumstances affect our sexual interest and arousal.

Let's talk about sex drive first, since it is more straightforward. Our sex drive is dynamic, and evolves with the hormonal changes in our lives. These hormonal changes in turn are triggered by life changes. For men, this can mean that their sex drive changes on a daily basis. Many men report that their sex drive is higher in the morn-ing. There is some recent evidence that men may go through a form of "menopause" sometime after their mid-to-late forties, in which their sex drive diminishes as they age. This makes scientific sense, because men's testosterone levels decrease as they age. In women, pregnancy, childbirth, and menopause (whether natural or surgically induced) alter levels of hormones, particularly testosterone, thus increasing or decreasing sex drive. Because birth control pills synthetically regulate hormone levels they affect sexual urges. A wonderful guide to the changes and cycles of desire in women is the book *Women, Sex, and Desire* by Elizabeth Davis.

Changes with Age

Does your sexual desire decline as you get older? There is some evidence that *sexual drive* declines in both men and women due to changes in testosterone in men and testosterone and estrogen in women. The fact that men tend to have less ejaculatory urgency as they age suggests this also. However, there is no direct evidence that I am aware of that suggests that a decline in sexual *desire* is a natural consequence of aging. There are many reasons why older people stop making love—a decrease in drive, illness, unavailability of a partner, unattractiveness of a partner—but loss of sexual desire is usually not one of these reasons.

If your sex drive has been strong in the past, it would be unusual for you to experience no desire to make love for a long period of time. If you are concerned that you have lost your sex drive (you never want to make love, even though you love your partner) and your surrounding conditions have not changed (you are not unduly stressed, are not on the Pill or other hormonal medications), there may be a biological cause for this. In this case, I recommend you consult an endocrinologist, who can check your hormone levels.

Sexual desire, on the other hand, is nourished by our mindset. So stress, lack of sexual confidence or experience, and mild depression can all have negative effects on our sexual desire. Low sexual desire is extremely common. In fact, in the 1980s so many people felt their desire succumb to stress and overwork that low sexual desire came to be known as the "yuppie disease." Luckily, in most cases low sexual desire can be easily remedied. If you feel this is what is affecting you, the exercises in this chapter and this book can help you relax, get comfortable with your sexual potential, and stir up your sexual desire.

A less common and more serious cause of low sexual desire is the repercussions of a traumatic event, particularly if it was of a sexual

nature. We often cope with trauma, whether recent or past, by disso-
ciating from the experience within ourselves. This can cause a number of problems that show up in an inability to have meaningful
sexual contact with another. If the trauma occurred when we were
children, the recollection of the traumatic event may remain inacces-
sible for a long time and only emerge later in life, causing great pain,
loss of sexual confidence, and confusion. If this is what you or your
partner are experiencing, I strongly urge you to seek professional coun-
seling so that you can learn to make love again. Putting this trauma
behind you will free you to embrace the full spectrum of your sexuality and the loving desire of your partner.

In my experience, sexual desire, especially in women, is an intricate interplay of factors. It has as much if not more to do with love,
acceptance, permission, body image, setting, and the attractiveness of
the partner as it does with hormones or stress levels. We have all been
in a situation where we didn't want to make love because we felt
unattractive, we were stressed out, our partner wasn't communicating
his feelings, the laundry wasn't done, or we were worried about the
kids or what we had to do the next day.

Psychological factors can affect a man's sexual desire also. Men
are particularly sensitive to concerns about their career and to compar-
isons with other men by their partner. Strangely, most sex researchers
have concentrated on studying men's sex drive rather than their
desire; the opposite is not true for women. We really don't know much
about the components that make up a man's sexual desire and the
factors that inhibit it.

So, what are the solutions, especially for women? If you have
certain conditions that need to be met before you make love, do your
best to create those conditions—up to a point. No setting can ever be
perfect, but if you like to make love in a beautiful setting with flowers, scents, music, linens, then create that setting, even if only for one
night. If you need to feel beautiful before you make love, set aside a
special time to take a bath, give yourself a manicure and pedicure, do

your hair, or put on a sexy outfit. All of these can boost your sexual desire because they nourish your feelings of sensuality.

What if you feel your sexual desire is low because of low self-esteem or poor body image? Explore the body image exercise from Chapter 4 by yourself. This can help you get in touch with your body's unique beauty and strengths. Make special efforts to look at yourself lovingly, without a critical eye. Do the body image exercise with your partner, then listen as he tells you what he loves and finds beautiful about your body.

What if your desire for your partner has waned or you don't find him or her as attractive as you used to? The bonding exercises in Chapter 2 will put you back in touch with your partner, the nuances of your intimate relationship, and the qualities that drew you to your partner. They may also help you realize aspects of each other that have grown and changed over time.

The Relationship between Sexual Desire and Your Behavior

Most people think that behavior follows desire. In other words, "we desire sex and so we make love." You could also say that sexual desire causes sexual behavior. But what most people don't realize is that behavior can also cause desire. Engaging in sexual activities that are very arousing can actually increase your desire, which in turn can influence your behavior. In other words, "we make love often, and it feels good, so we desire sex more often."

Based on the fact that sexual behavior can increase desire, most of the exercises in this book will help you feel more sexual desire. Don't be put off from doing them because you think, "I just don't feel like it tonight." You don't need any particular level of sexual desire to do any of the exercises in this book. All you need is the loving mind-set and a willingness to spend time with your partner.

If you would like to increase your sexual desire, spend a few weeks doing the bonding exercises in Chapter 2 and the touching exercises in Chapter 3. Make dates with each other (or yourself) to do them a few times each week. Pay special attention to the peaking exercise, as it can really increase your desire levels along with your endorphin levels. Then do the partner exercises in Chapter 6 and the intercourse exercises in Chapter 7, again with special emphasis on peaking. Lastly, try the advanced techniques below for making love better.

♀ Exercise ♂
The Silent Caress

Begin by sharing a slow, focused front caress with your partner. Then concentrate your caress on one area of your partner's body. Choose an area that is physically bothering your partner, or one that you feel you don't pay enough attention to. You could also choose the genitals as an area you would like to caress if you wish.

Let's say that you have chosen your partner's abdomen as the focus of your caress. Caress the abdomen in the usual sensate focus way, and then move your hand away so it is not quite touching the skin, but is so close that you can feel the energy flow between you. I like to think of this energy you feel as the energy of desire. Alternate between actually lightly touching your partner and not touching, so that you can barely tell if you are touching or not. Pour your attention and all your loving intention into your hand. You can use this caress on any part of the body.

♀ Exercise ♂
From the Heart

Caress the front of your partner's body with one hand. With loving intention place your other hand lightly over your partner's heart. Do a nontouching caress over your partner's heart as you caress the rest of his or her body. You may also want to try lightly placing your ear over your partner's heart during the caress.

. . .

Are your lives very hectic or busy? Do you and your partner often feel you hardly have time together, because one of you is coming when the other is going? Here are some very advanced exercises to help you both feel you are on the same road, traveling in the same direction. They call on the peaking and plateauing techniques you have learned earlier, and create incredible feelings of connected energy. And as you men over forty may have realized by now, it's often easier to practice peaking and plateauing at this age because the need to come, and come soon, is less intense.

♀ Exercise ♂
Mutual Orgasm

I am sure you have heard the phrase "simultaneous orgasm," in reference to a couple having an orgasm at the same time during intercourse. In sexology, for a long time simultaneous orgasm was touted as the be-all and end-all of lovemaking. It eventually fell out of favor with sex therapists because many of them realized this point of view put too much pressure on couples, especially men who have difficulty with premature ejaculation problems and women who have difficulty reaching orgasm during intercourse.

Some of us, however, have not given up on the rare potential of simultaneous orgasm—which I prefer to call "mutual orgasm" because it suggests so much more than simply two orgasms happening at the same time. "Mutual orgasm" also reflects the idea that each lover enjoys their partner's orgasm as well as his or her own. With the techniques in this book, especially peaking and plateauing, you and your partner can learn so much about each other's arousal and sexual response, as well as how to gauge your own, that you will be able to enjoy mutual orgasms.

The Exercise Mutual orgasm is an outgrowth of the sensate focus intercourse from Chapter 7. You begin with some unstructured foreplay or focusing caresses to awaken your senses. Then decide who will be on top. Bring your bodies together in an intercourse position in which you are face to face. Whoever is on top controls the speed of the thrusting and should start as slowly as possible. The partner on the bottom should respond, moving in tandem.

As you roll through slow, sensuous thrusting, peak together up through gentle and strong levels of arousal. Relax, breathe, and focus on the sensations in your penis and vagina. Men, think of yourself as caressing your partner's vagina with your penis. Women, think of yourself as caressing your partner's penis with the walls of your vagina. Keep your motion shared and mutual as you thrust together and slide apart. Look at each other as you move.

If you have done many peaking and plateauing exercises, you are probably very aware of your own and your partner's arousal levels. Remember that the best cues for your partner's arousal level are heart rate and breathing.

When the person on top climbs to the brink of orgasm, the other should be at a point to follow. As you plunge into orgasm, take a deep breath, relax your body, open your eyes wide, and look into your partner's eyes. With practice you will find that you have the ability either to hold back slightly until your partner is ready or to accelerate your arousal slightly to match your partner's.

If you frequently experience mutual orgasm with your partner you may think this is as good as lovemaking gets. But what if you could experience multiple orgasms together? Read on!

♀ Exercise ♂
Multiple Orgasms for Men

In *How to Make Love All Night* I wrote extensively about how men can master this delicious experience, but I would like to explain the basics of it here again. For a couple it can really be the icing on the cake, so to speak, of mutual orgasm.

Contrary to popular belief, it *is* possible for men to have multiple orgasms the way that women do. To learn how, you first need to understand that orgasm and ejaculation are really two different body processes. An orgasm is a full-body response that includes spasms of the long muscles of the body, an elevated heart rate, rapid breathing, and an intense feeling of pleasure and release. Ejaculation is a localized genital phenomenon that occurs when the PC muscle spasms and forces semen out of the penis.

Every man can become multiply orgasmic by learning to let his body carry over into the sensations of orgasm while delaying or withholding ejaculation. He can do this by being intensely aware of the sensations that happen right at the point of ejaculatory inevitability or the "point of no return," and keeping himself from going over that point. Because he doesn't ejaculate he can maintain an erection and continue making love, during which time he may go on to have another or several more orgasms. Many men especially enjoy ejaculating with their final orgasm.

Becoming multiply orgasmic holds several benefits for men. By understanding the powers of orgasmic potential you gain insight into your partner's response and it becomes easier for the two of you to communicate about sexual matters. In becoming multiply orgasmic, you learn to prolong and savor the sexual pleasures of lovemaking. You may also increase your ability to give pleasure to your partner. Many men experience deep, altered states of consciousness. And women whose partners become multiply orgasmic often delight in the sharing of this very special experience.

The Exercise   There are numerous, detailed exercises in *How to Make Love All Night*, but you can begin with the preliminary exercise here. Some men have learned this in just a few sessions.

First, try bringing yourself to orgasmic potential alone a couple of times before trying it with your partner. Begin with a sensual genital caress. Peak yourself two or three times through increasingly stronger levels of arousal. When you reach an urgent level, practice plateauing once or twice. At that split-second before your PC muscle starts to spasm at the point of inevitability, squeeze your PC muscle as tight as you can for five to ten seconds, open your eyes, take a few deep breaths, and relax all your other muscles. You will have an unusual sensation in which you have an orgasm but don't ejaculate. If you ejaculate a little bit, it just means you need to practice your timing.

When you try the same exercise when making love with your partner, focus very hard on your arousal and on sustaining your plateaus. Many men prefer doing this from the kneeling position because it naturally relaxes most of the muscles in your body, but you should find a position that is comfortable for you. Use as many pillows and cushions as you need. I have also found that the men who learn this the most quickly are those who are able to get away from a performance attitude and make love just because they enjoy it and love making love with their partners.

♀ Exercise ♂
Multiple Orgasms for Women

For women, the way to trigger multiple orgasms is similar to the plateauing with intercourse exercise from Chapter 7. Multiple orgasms may be very strong or very quiet, somewhere in-between, or a combination of all three. For some women the first orgasm they have during a lovemaking session is the strongest, and the later orgasms are like smaller "aftershocks." For other women, all orgasms are created equal. For yet others the first orgasms in a lovemaking session are small and genitally focused, but they get stronger, involve more and more of the body, and build to an explosive climax. You can use the peaking and plateauing techniques as indicated below to help you discover which pattern works best for you individually.

You can have multiple orgasms in any position. Many women find that being on top is more active and gives them more ability to control their stroking and arousal. Other women find that having their partners kneel between their legs while they lie on their back provides more stimulation, particularly to their G-spot. I encourage you to try different positions and different types of orgasms. You may first want to try multiple orgasms alone with genital caresses or using a dildo or sexual aid, before trying them with your partner.

The Exercise   Begin by relaxing fully, and making sure you are well lubricated. Bring yourself to two or three peaks at increasingly stronger levels of arousal. Then plateau at an urgent level of arousal, using breathing, pelvic movements, a PC squeeze, or by switching focus. When you reach peaks at a very urgent level of arousal, instead of plateauing again let yourself wash over into an orgasm. Then continue stimulation and peaking until you reach another orgasm. The more you are able to let yourself go and embrace the full spectrum of your bodily sensations, the more likely you will be to have multiple orgasms.

Some women have difficulty stimulating themselves again directly after orgasm because their genitals (especially the clitoris) become too sensitive. What I have found in my experience and in my clinical practice is that you are less likely to experience this hypersensitivity if you allow your arousal to climb and then really subside in the peaking pattern. You might also want to experiment with different types of stimulation to different parts of your genitals.

When you feel ready, begin trying these patterns in lovemaking sessions with your partner. As you increase your orgasmic potential, I'll bet you and your partner increase your desire for sex and your desire for each other as well.

Chapter 10
Loving Words

Y ou may be surprised that I have waited this long to talk about, well...talking. I did this purposely, because I believe that learning to make love better than ever means starting from the ground up. In a sense, by learning how to bond, how to touch yourself, how to touch your partner, and how to convey love during intercourse, you have learned how to deconstruct your sex life and build it back up again. And make it stronger than ever.

In each of the foregoing chapters I have shown you a new element to add to your loving with your partner. For example, you learned the sensate focus process with yourself before you attempted it with a partner, then with your partner you learned how to deal with nonverbal performance pressure. Now it is time to add verbal communication to your lovemaking repertoire. If there is one clear idea that I hope you get out of this chapter, it is that communicating about lovemaking need not be awkward or demanding. It can be straightforward and pressure-free—and freeing. As we get older, it becomes easier for us to communicate about things that were difficult to talk about when we were younger. Maybe then they mattered too much, or we felt we were different and no one would understand, or we were told sex was taboo and "dirty." Now that we have become more trusting in our relationships, we realize that everyone *is* different but we're also all the same, and maybe we see that sex is a pure opportunity to create something beautiful and fulfilling. Crossing forty may cost us some of our primal vigor, but it brings its gifts.

One of these gifts, which can enrich and deepen your emotional relationship, is to learn to talk to each other more comfortably and unabashedly about making love. And talking about lovemaking need not be clinical or prescriptive. To learn some fun, sexy word games try the exercises in my book *Talk Sexy to the One You Love*. But if you feel a little shy with your partner, or are in a verbally awkward relationship, try this basic exercise.

♀ Exercise ♂
Observe, Reflect, Ask

This is an exercise that is often used by therapists trying to help couples improve their communication. In this version it is adapted for use during lovemaking.

A lot of couples, regardless of how long they have been together, do fabulously with the touching and non-verbal aspects of the sensate focus exercises but freeze up when trying to communicate verbally during lovemaking. Yet being able to express your intimacy in words can bring you and your partner great pleasure, both physical and emotional. I especially encourage those of you who are able to communicate well with your partner most of the time but have a difficult time saying anything during sex to try this helpful exercise.

The Exercise   As usual, one of you will be active while the other is passive. Decide together what caresses the active person will do, choosing those that do not make the passive partner anxious or likely to withdraw.

The active partner should caress for about half an hour, going from a back caress to a front caress, to a genital caress, to sensuous oral sex. As the passive partner, stop your partner at some point in the exercise when you are really enjoying what is going on. First, observe to yourself, "She's stroking my penis in a way that I find really pleasurable." Then reflect that thought to your partner, saying it out loud as an "I" statement: "I really like the way you are caressing my penis." Then ask your partner to continue that caress for a few minutes: "Please caress my penis this way for a few more minutes."

During the half-hour exercise, observe and ask for several different things. Then switch roles. When you are finished, embrace each other and ground yourselves, then reflect on how talking during lovemaking made you feel.

♀ Exercise ♂
Genital Caress with Verbal Feedback

Remember the genital caress you did with your partner in Chapter 6? At that point when you were starting it was important that the exercise was pressure-free, with no verbal communication. But now, in order to learn more about each other's response, you and your partner should try a version of the genital caress in which you give each other feedback about the type of touch you enjoy on your genitals.

The Exercise   Decide who will be the active partner and who the passive. As part of your attempt to achieve clearer communication, you and your partner could try to make this simple decision in a way and using words that feel comfortable and clear to both of you. Try to say what you want without anticipating each other's response or preference, in a way that shows your respect for the other and leaves room for disagreement and resolution. It is a small thing, and both of you know that whoever goes first, the other will get his or her turn. But being a little more aware while making this simple decision can model better communication between you. It establishes a healthy pattern of asking for what you want in your sexual loving interactions, and you can use that pattern in all the exercises you do after this one.

Begin by doing a sensuous genital caress with manual or oral stimulation or both. When you are passive, at the end of the caress tell your partner one or two things that he or she did that you found particularly pleasurable. Be specific, for example, "I really liked it when you stroked the length of my labia slowly." Then ask your partner to do those things again. Allow yourself to enjoy what you asked for for several minutes. If it is not exactly what you wanted, gently guide your partner's hand or face and give him or her more feedback until the caress is exactly the way it pleases you. Then tell your partner something that you would like that he or she didn't do. You may take your partner's hand and gently guide it to receive what you want for a few minutes.

Try not to phrase things negatively. Instead of "I didn't like the way you pressed so hard on my clitoris," you might say "I like my clitoris stroked and rubbed but not hard or long, and maybe you could finger me in between." The point of the exercise is not to critique your partner, which creates alienation and defensiveness, but to share with your partner the types of touch you enjoy, and give your partner an opportunity to experience the pleasure of really arousing you.

♀ Exercise ♂
Asking for What You Want

One of the great myths that we seem to be born believing is that sexual expression comes naturally, and so sexual pleasures should come naturally as well. While this may be the case for a lucky few, for most of us nothing could be further from the truth. Most people develop far more satisfaction and intimacy in their sexual relationship when they begin to communicate their feelings specifically and clearly with their partner. "Asking for What You Want" is a communication exercise that helps you feel comfortable asking for what you want in a pressure-free way. But be careful what you ask for—you'll get it! So enjoy it!

The Exercise   This exercise begins the minute the two of you enter the bedroom. Mutually decide who will be active first. Let's say in this case it is the man. From the moment he enters the room, he asks for anything he wants. Nothing in the exercise will happen unless he requests it. If he wants his partner to be naked, he must say, "Please take off your clothes." If he wishes his partner to remove his clothes, he must say, "Please take off my clothes." And so on.

Make sure you tell your partner everything that you want her to do. You may ask for anything you can think of or desire, but you need to be specific. If what your partner does is not exactly what you desire, say so kindly, and give her directions until she gets it right. Feel free to enjoy whatever you have asked your partner to do for as long as you want. Unless you have achieved a really strong level of mutuality and commitment between you, at this stage of the program only ask your partner for things that you have done together in the past, and only ask for things you are both comfortable with. If you repeat the exercise later, you can ask for more.

As the active, asking partner you may also do whatever you like, as long as you tell your partner what you are going to do beforehand. For example, if you would like to touch her for a while, you could say, "I want you to lie down so I can caress your back for a while."

When you are the passive partner in this exercise, simply do as your partner asks. Don't worry—you will have your turn too! Much as you might want to initiate something, don't. See if you can actually do what is asked for your own enjoyment and focus on it. The secret is to accommodate your partner's wishes while still enjoying the activities for yourself. However, don't agree to do anything that you find painful or unpleasant.

Some people find this exercise awkward and even difficult because they are not used to asking for what they want, or giving in to their partner. When you are the asker, be assertive and don't settle for something other than what you desire. Make your requests clear. For example, rather than saying, "Would you like to give me a front caress?" say, "Please give me a front caress" or, "I'd like you to give me a front caress." Remember, too, that if your partner says no to something you request it doesn't mean, "No, never, that's disgusting." It simply means, "No, I don't want to do that particular activity right now."

Try this exercise initially with each person in the active role for half an hour. The exercise can be stressful, but it can also pinpoint problems you may be having in asserting or enjoying yourself. Were you paralyzed by thoughts such as "I wanted to ask for such-and-such but I didn't think you'd want to do it?" Did you feel on an equal footing? Did you find it difficult to be clear, and explain what you wanted? If you had these or other thoughts, share them with your partner and try the exercise again at some later time.

The major benefit of this exercise is that you learn to ask for sensual or sexual pleasure in a healthy, pressure-free, loving way. As a result you and your partner will reduce the second-guessing in your sexual communication.

In order to make love better than ever you must also feel comfortable with your body. You will also be able to experience greater sexual pleasure if you are comfortable discussing your body with your partner. The following two exercises are designed to help you do just that.

♀ Exercise ♂
Body Image—Nonverbal

Think of this as a sensate focus exercise using the eyes instead of the hands. This exercise is a prelude to the following one, in which you and your partner discuss feelings about your bodies. Most couples find it more comfortable to do a preliminary exercise first, in which you both become comfortable having your partner gaze at you while you are nude.

The Exercise　The room should be well lit, and have a large mirror, preferably full-length. First, take off all of your clothes, stand a few feet apart, and gaze at each other silently for a minute. Look warmly into each other's eyes, then slowly and appreciatively take in your partner's facial features. Notice things that you have never noticed before or things that you haven't taken the time to notice in a while.

Next, both of you should lower your gaze to take in your partner's torso. Let your eyes move slowly over his or her body, as if in a caress. Take your time and look on each body part for as long as it takes to visually enjoy it. Now mutually shift your gaze downward over the abdomen and legs. Take time to look at each other's genitals. Then each partner should turn around so that the other person can look at the back of his or her body. Again start at the top, the head and the neck, and slowly move your gaze downward over the back, the buttocks, thighs and knees, the calves, ankles and heels. If you have seen your partner's body naked many times before, use this exercise to appreciate, rather than to see for the first time. If you find your attention wandering, silently tell yourself something specially attractive, arousing, or interesting about the part of your partner's body you are looking at.

Even if you have seen each other nude many times it may not have been acceptable in your relationship to stare at certain body parts, such as the breasts or genitals. You may be in the habit of wearing sleepwear to bed, and sexual activity may take place only with the lights off. You may not be able to walk around the house nude because you have children at home, or are looking after a parent or parents. For whatever reason, you may not have much experience seeing your partner nude or being seen in the nude, so take this opportunity to look openly, frankly, and appreciatively at your partner's nude body.

Your nudity may cause you some anxiety. Bear in mind that your partner may feel the same. If you feel anxious or self-conscious during this part of the exercise, take some deep breaths and express the fact that you feel anxiety to your partner. Men and women usually have different anxieties about their bodies and about being nude in front of a partner.

For a man, the two common anxieties are a fear that his penis is too small (every male client I ever worked with expressed concern during this exercise that his penis was not large enough) and concerns about having or not having an erection. Men have different ideas about how long it should take them to get an erection when they are naked with a woman. Some expect to have an erection immediately; others may allow themselves one minute or five minutes. Others think that they should not have an erection at all and are embarrassed if they do have one.

The body image exercise is not a sexual exercise. If you do have an erection during the exercise, just enjoy it and keep doing the exercise. Don't try to make your erection harder, and don't try to make it go away. It is perfectly normal to either have or not have an erection during this exercise.

While men's anxieties tend to be about their genitals, women tend to worry about being overweight, and about whether their partner will find some of their body parts unacceptable. Most women tend to think that their breasts are too small or too saggy, and that their hips and thighs are too wide. Part of their reason for feeling overweight is that our culture and society place a totally unwarranted—and unhealthy—emphasis on slimness, idealizing a body that is unattainable for the vast majority of women. Hopefully, doing this exercise (and all of the exercises in this book) will help you to accept your body more.

As we get older, men tend to worry about graying, about losing hair, about getting flabby and developing jowls. Women tend to worry even more about putting on weight, about developing wrinkles, and about their breasts drooping. Sometimes it helps to know that we all feel these insecurities; we can admit them and even share them, get real, and move on. Another thing I like to do with clients who have these concerns is to suggest they visit a health club and note who they feel more drawn to: the attractive but self-involved people pumping iron or doing advanced jazzercise in tight leotards, or the ones enjoying their workout, smiling at you, sharing the good energy and pleasure of being there with the others in the room. Hard bodies may be fun in fantasies, but sexual fulfillment is about a shared capacity for arousal, openness to energy, and a willingness to connect.

If you do feel anxious about whether your partner finds your body attractive, just accept the fact that you have these feelings for now. Remember that doing the body image exercises and all of the other exercises in this book does not require a body that meets certain standards of attractiveness. What matters is the loving sexual connection you make with your partner.

Your anxieties and feelings about your body and about your partner's reaction to it are real. The body image exercise will help you learn to accept the negative feelings about your body and learn not to let these feelings get in the way of your enjoyment. The exercise will help you learn to relax when you are nude. It will also help you recognize that nudity is a natural state that is not necessarily sexual.

♀ Exercise ♂
Body Image—Verbal

Do you remember the nonverbal body image exercise in Chapter 4 in which you practiced loving your body? Here you will share some of that self-love with your partner by describing your body to him or her. In this next body image exercise one of you is passive while the other is active. You will need a hand-held mirror for this.

The Exercise When you are active, look at yourself in the mirror carefully, using a hand mirror to examine the back of your body, then talk about it with your partner. Let's say that the woman decides to be active first. She takes a long look at herself in the mirror and describes all the parts of her body, and her feelings associated with each part, while the man sits comfortably and watches and listens.

Start with your hair and say what you like or dislike about it, describe good or bad feelings or memories that are associated with it, and say whether you like to touch it or have it touched, and how that feels. Then do the same for the rest of your body: face, neck, shoulders, back, breasts, arms, hands, stomach, thighs, buttocks, genitals, legs, feet. You may want to talk about your height, weight, body hair, and any characteristics such as moles, birthmarks, or scars.

After this, consider your body as a whole, and tell your partner your favorite and least favorite parts. What do you consider your best and worst features? What parts cause you anxiety? What parts don't you like to have touched and looked at, and why? What would you change if you could change anything about your body? What would you like to look like and why? You might touch and stroke yourself as you do this part—touching or stroking a body part can bring up memories.

If you are the passive partner, you may agree or disagree with your partner's descriptions—but remain quiet. Don't interrupt, make comments, or ask questions; you will exchange feedback at the end of the exercise. For each partner—both active and passive—things will come up that you could not have predicted.

After you have switched roles and the other person has described his or her body, discuss the following: Did you feel that your partner was realistic about his or her body? Why? Which part of your partner's body do you especially like? Be careful not to negate your partner's feelings when you phrase your thoughts. When your partner describes his or her feelings about your body, listen carefully. Believe and accept them, even though they may not coincide with your opinions.

Remember that flattery isn't loving, but honesty is. The best-looking people don't always have the best body images. Also remember that this is not a time for bringing up negative or critical feelings about your partner, or about your past or current relationship. This is a time to learn how you and your partner feel about your own bodies and to honor yourselves in preparation for learning to show your love for each other in more sexual ways.

If you find this exercise uncomfortable, there are options that can make it easier. If you are anxious about appearing completely nude in front of your partner, start with just part of your clothing off. You may find that if you go into a lot of detail about each body part, this exercise will take a long time. You might want to get together once a day with your partner for fifteen minutes or so for a week, instead of trying to do the whole body all at once.

The body image exercises are not easy, because we don't usually discuss our feelings about our bodies with other people. Exploring these issues together will build trust between you and your partner. It will give you practice in communicating about feelings. And it will provide information about how your partner feels about his or her body and, by extension, sexuality and lovemaking in general.

Another purpose of the body image exercise is to find out if you and your partner have realistic views of your bodies. As a woman, you may find your body unattractive and think your partner is not telling the truth when he says that he likes your breasts or your thighs. If you are a man, you may feel that your penis is too small, when in fact your partner likes the way it looks and feels. These feelings about yourself and the way you look are probably not negative enough to stand in the way of doing sensate focus exercises together or making love, but they keep you from realizing your true potential. When a person's body image is either totally unrealistic or so negative that he or she cannot relax enough to enjoy sensual arousal, problems do arise.

Many people with unrealistic body images are good-looking, but their self-esteem is so low that they consider themselves ugly. As a surrogate partner I worked with clients of all levels of relative attractiveness. Not once did I encounter a client physically unattractive enough for it to interfere with our ability to engage in sensate focus exercises. Both attractive and unattractive bodies feel good to touch.

However, if there is some aspect of your appearance that you would like to change and realistically could, there are a number of excellent books and other resources available on skin care, health, exercise, and clothing choice. Motivation will help you do this, and looking more attractive can boost your self-esteem and can show your partner that you respect yourself and care about your health.

In addition to all of the above, just getting feelings and anxieties about your bodies out in the open can eliminate further negative experiences. You may also learn that your partner's reaction to being touched may have much less to do with the way you touch than with his or her own anxieties about body image or body memories.

Have you or your partner had a traumatic experience that has caused you to feel uncomfortable about your naked body or embarrassed about a certain body part? If this exercise brings up a powerful issue for you, remember that just getting it out in the open can help to release it. When dealing with any powerful traumatic memory, such as one of physical or sexual abuse, I encourage you to seek the assistance of a qualified therapist to help you deal with the issue completely. If a traumatic memory comes up for your partner, accept his or her feelings completely and be very supportive.

* * *

It is now time to switch gears from the body image and move to a couple more exercises that can help you share new levels of verbal intimacy with your partner. The next exercise is similar to the switch focus exercise you did by yourself in Chapter 5. Now you will share it with your partner.

♀ Exercise ♂
Mutual Switch Focus

Remember that there are a number of things that you can focus on when you make love. The basic sensate focus caresses teach you to focus on one body part at a time. When you learned to switch focus by yourself in Chapter 5, you learned that you could add depth to a simple sensate focus exercise by either focusing on the body part you were touching or focusing on the feeling of the hand touching the body part.

When you do a switch focus exercise with your partner, the possibilities are multiplied. If one person is active and the other is passive, you can focus on your hand touching your partner's body, or on the part of his or her body that you are touching. If you are both caressing each other at the same time, you can focus on your hand touching your partner's body, your partner's body being touched by your hand, your partner's hand touching your body, or your body being touched by your partner's hand.

This switch focus exercise will help you develop your sensate focus abilities. It will also help you learn to communicate better verbally, as one of you will give the instructions throughout the exercise.

The Exercise Begin with spoon breathing and tender focusing caresses, then position yourselves in a comfortable side-by-side position so that you can caress each other's genitals with one hand. You will do this simultaneously throughout the exercise.

When you begin the mutual caress, both of you should focus on the man's genitals. Then after several minutes switch your focus to the woman's genitals. For the next switch, concentrate on the man's hand. For the last switch, focus on the woman's hand. Remember to breathe and relax also. Take five or more minutes between switches, to give yourselves the time to focus and enjoy the caress.

This exercise is not easy! It takes concentration and self-discipline to focus on all of these different perspectives. It may help if one person decides when to switch the focus, and says out loud, "Now, let's both focus on your genitals," for example.

Spend about fifteen to twenty minutes doing this exercise. This will allow for several switches. After you have focused on all four possibilities, try combining sensations. For example, say, "Let's both focus on my hand touching your genitals at the same time." You could also see if you can both focus on everything that is happening the same way you focus on the total sound of an orchestra rather than on individual instruments.

This switch focus technique also works during mutual oral sex. A lot of people don't like mutual oral sex because it is harder to focus on your own pleasure. Using this switch focus technique can help you to learn to concentrate on any one sensation for a while so that you can enjoy it to the fullest.

♀ Exercise ♂
Fantasy Sharing with Mutual Masturbation

A fantasy is normally a private mental experience that an individual finds sexually stimulating, and it could be about actual sexual activity or it could be sensual. Sharing fantasies with a partner can be one of the most verbally intimate things you do together. In fact, many people have fantasies about sharing fantasies! Fantasy sharing can also be done if you have some temporary limitation on your lovemaking, perhaps due to illness or due to distance. I know of a couple who does this regularly over the phone when one of them is away on business.

The Exercise   One of you is active while the other is passive; the active partner relates his or her fantasy. Lie next to each other on or in your bed. Lie on your backs if that is comfortable for you (use pillow supports if you need them).

The active person will begin by describing a fantasy. This could be a fantasy made up as you go along, or a recurring fantasy that has the power to stimulate you. The fantasy could be about your partner or about someone you know—or don't know.

If you have difficulties jump-starting your ability to story-tell, describe your fantasy with as much attention to the five senses as you can. For example, describe smells, tastes, sounds, and textures. Try to really evoke the setting. Alternatively, you can picture yourself in a scene from an erotic movie you have seen or an erotic book you have read. Describe what you remember from the book or movie in detail, but make yourself the main character.

It may be embarrassing for you to contemplate your partner's reaction to a particular fantasy. That is why sometimes it is easiest to build your ability to fantasize from the ground up by beginning with the above suggestions. One thing that can help is to describe the fantasy as if it happened in a dream.

You can add an extra exciting dimension to fantasy sharing if you both masturbate. You can do this a number of ways. One person can share a fantasy and masturbate while the other watches and listens. Or one person can share a fantasy while the other listens and masturbates. Alternatively, one of you can share a fantasy while both of you masturbate. You can even share a fantasy while masturbating your partner, who can then lie back and revel in both your story and your touch. When you do this be sure to allow time so that both of you can share a fantasy.

♀ Exercise ♂
A New Way of Talking

I hardly ever hear people say positive things about their partners anymore, and it is an absolute shame. Perhaps as a society we have all fallen out of the habit. Perhaps we tend to value the negative in conversations too much. Maybe we don't realize the power of positive thought.

This exercise is an ongoing one, and the more it finds its way into your day-to-day life, the better. First, become aware of whether you tend to talk with, at, or about your partner. When you are talking with your partner, make sure you are talking with your partner and not to or at him or her.

Second, resolve to say something good about your partner to another person at least once a day. This good thing can be as simple as, "My wife is really great. She makes me laugh all the time," or "You won't believe what my husband did last night. It made me so happy."

As a part of this exercise, why not try to do something nice for your partner that is sure to inspire this type of thought or comment on his or her part?

Chapter 11
Loving Men

Although the focus in *Making Love Better Than Ever* is on the loving power of sexuality, I have included two extensive chapters on making love if you have sexual concerns or problems. This chapter deals with making love with a man who has sexual concerns or problems, and the next chapter deals with making love with a woman who has sexual concerns or problems.

More importantly, these two chapters deal with making love if you are a man or woman whose partner has sexual concerns. It is important that women and men understand and support their partners if the latter have sexual concerns. So much is known and easily understood today about sexual problems, and there is so much that partners can do to help each other, that it is no longer acceptable to remain uninformed. For that reason most of this chapter about men is written for their female partner, just as most of the next chapter about women is addressed to their male partner.

The first thing your partner should understand is that sexual concerns and problems are extremely common. In some ways, the fact that sexual problems are often stigmatized is really a hoax, one that seems to be played by everyone on everyone for the benefit of no one. All that is achieved is that many people, women and men, become trapped in isolation, avoidance, or self-blame. I have a soft spot for the Sixties because I think this is what people—at least some people—meant then when they said that sex should be free. Not that we should all feel free to sleep with everyone and use each other for sexual gratification in uninvolved, narcissistic, and eventually unsatisfying ways, but that sex should be free of these conspiracies of silence, guilt, and competitive posturing.

If your partner has a sexual concern or problem, there may be times when you feel that he doesn't want to make love at all. Or you may think your partner doesn't want to make love with you. I have included these two chapters to reassure you that you can find a way to make love and express your loving connection even if you both have had doubts about your ability to do so.

The information in this chapter covers the most common concerns that men have about their sexuality. It also includes specific single and couple exercises that will allow you to actually treat a problem together by making love in the sensate focus manner.

The most common male sexual concerns are ejaculating too fast, losing erections, and not being able to ejaculate. I'll address each concern separately and provide several exercises that can be beneficial for them.

Satisfying Ejaculations

Premature ejaculation is the clinical name for the condition in which a man feels he ejaculates too quickly. Premature ejaculation is not defined by how long a man lasts (whether in seconds or minutes), how many strokes he can make before ejaculation, or whether you have an orgasm when he makes love with you. Rather, an ejaculation is considered premature if it happens before the man wishes, or when he doesn't feel in control of his ejaculation.

Some experts believe that it doesn't matter how long a man is able to last in intercourse before he ejaculates. Their idea is that if he ejaculates before he wants to he can simply continue intercourse with a flaccid penis. After spending many years working with men who want better ejaculatory control when making love with their partners, I get upset when I read these ideas. The time a man lasts during lovemaking can affect his opportunity to experience loving contact with his partner. Most men want to last longer so that they can experience their partner's loving touch and share mutual arousal for a longer time. Premature ejaculation can be a serious hindrance to your partner's enjoyment of your lovemaking, his ability to feel and express intimacy, not to mention his self-esteem, if it detracts from his ability to show you love and accept your love.

That said, I do agree that the quality of lovemaking is not dependent on the amount of time the two of you spend in intercourse or the amount of your activity. I believe in ejaculation control for life rather than making love for a certain amount of time. Sometimes the two of you may want to spend long periods of time in the types of loving intercourse described in Chapter 7. At other times you may just want a quickie. Both options celebrate your intimacy, so you should be able to enjoy them but you won't if your partner has concerns about rapid ejaculation.

For your partner, ejaculating before he wants to can actually be an easy concern to deal with, especially when you are willing to help.

Since premature ejaculation occurs when the PC muscle spasms out of control, the PC muscle exercises and relaxation exercises in this book are a must. All of the sensate focus caresses in this book—both those that he does by himself and those that you do together—will help him learn to last longer as they help him pay attention to his sensations instead of ignoring them. The peaking process will also help him learn to recognize his arousal levels. During exercises such as the genital caress, peaking and plateauing, encourage your partner not to worry about ejaculating. Tell him not to hold back. If he ejaculates during one of the exercises before he wants to, both of you should just enjoy it. If he would like still more practice with techniques to help him last longer, you can try the following two exercises. When you do these exercises make sure to start them with relaxing spoon breathing and focusing caresses, and approach them with a loving mindset rather than a performance orientation.

♀ Exercise ♂
Peaking with the PC Squeeze

Learning to use your PC muscle to put the brakes on your arousal is a little tricky. Normally, if you reach a certain level of arousal and then quickly squeeze the PC muscle once or twice, your arousal will go down a level. This takes a little time to learn because there are several different ways to squeeze. Your partner may have to experiment a little bit to see which one works best for him. He should work on this by himself first before trying it with you.

There are three basic patterns of PC muscle squeezes: one long hard squeeze, two medium squeezes, or several quick squeezes in a row, similar to the PC muscle spasms during ejaculation.

Your partner begins this exercise on his own with a genital caress and some peaks. During the peaks, he will try different PC squeezes. The goal is to find the smallest PC squeeze that takes his arousal down a level without affecting his erection. If he squeezes his PC muscle too much before he has a full erection he may temporarily lose it, but it will come back in a few minutes.

The Exercise   Your partner uses arousal awareness to find the best PC squeeze for him. As he peaks through stronger and then urgent arousal levels, he focuses on recognizing his arousal level as he squeezes his PC muscle. At the point of inevitability, he lets go in an orgasm without trying to hold back. He should repeat this exercise on two or three different days, then the two of you can try it together.

As A Couple   Give your partner front and genital caresses to inspire his arousal. As he begins to peak, ask him his arousal level, after which he'll squeeze his PC muscle in his preferred way. Caress him through arousal peaks. At each peak, after he squeezes, both of you relax. Continue peaking and see if he can use his PC to lower his arousal even at an urgent level. He can let go into an orgasm and ejaculate if he wishes.

Once you have done this exercise together you are ready for intercourse. This first time you make love, do it in the very specific way described below. After that, indulge in intercourse peaking and plateauing as described in Chapter 7.

♀ Exercise ♂
First Intercourse for Premature Ejaculation

Before You Begin   Using hand and oral stimulation, bring your partner to strong peaks. Then lie on your sides facing each other, with your legs interwoven so that your genitals are up against each other. This is a comfortable position in which neither person is on top supporting their weight on their arms.

The Exercise   Stroke a lot of lubrication on your partner's penis and around your vagina. Now slowly insert his penis, whether it is flaccid, erect, or somewhere in between, into your vagina. Both of you relax all your muscles and breathe, while he notes his arousal level. If it is gentle or just barely strong, he should begin slow pelvic rolls and thrusts and start peaking. He should peak at stronger and stronger levels a few times, stopping in between for as long as he needs, trying to do several peaks for about fifteen minutes. Then, if he wants, he can ejaculate.

If your partner's arousal level is strong when you first insert his penis, have him withdraw and allow it to go down, then he can re-enter you (even if he is flaccid). If all he is able to do this first time is lie inside you without moving, that's fine—it is progress! Enjoy the sexual intimacy it brings. You can keep repeating this exercise until your partner can recognize his arousal levels and move inside you comfortably.

After you are both comfortable doing this side-to-side position for fifteen minutes, you can try the peaking exercise in different positions, as described in Chapter 7. The only difference between your partner and someone not concerned with ejaculation is that you may have to move a little slower, repeat exercises, or have him use his PC muscle for some peaks.

Satisfying Erections

This is a big area of concern for men and an area in which loving is really needed. Men spend too much time concerned about the hardness of their erections rather than the loving feelings they have for their partner or that their partner has for them. Women want to make love to a man, not a penis.

Unfortunately, the medical community often contributes to this unhealthy attitude. The biggest breakthroughs in treating sexual problems in the past few years have been medical, including drugs, penile implants, vacuum pumps to create erections, and penile injections. I believe the medical community does men a disservice by convincing them that most erection problems are physical. This tendency to view our bodies as machines that need fixing ultimately stands in the way of lovemaking, because we are our minds *and* bodies, and we just don't work that way. I am not against medical solutions for men who have irreversible physical erection problems. For those men, medical solutions can often make the difference between being able to express sexual love to their partners and not being able to. However, sometimes medical solutions—when they are improperly recommended—can interfere with the intimacy that occurs during lovemaking.

What Is a "Normal" Erection?

Erections reflect the state of a man's physical and psychological health. Erection problems can have various causes, including medical conditions, stress, and relationship problems. While most men consider erections an all-or-nothing phenomenon (either you have one or you don't), this is not true. A man can have a partial erection and still make love. A man can have a completely flaccid penis and still make love. And no matter the hardness of his erection, he can experience every level of arousal through orgasm.

For the purpose of understanding more about erections, think of them on a scale from one to ten. This is different from the arousal scale you used during the peaking exercises. Here we are concerned with how *hard* your partner's erection is, not what he is feeling. On the erection scale, level one is no erection—a completely flaccid penis. Levels two through four are what are called filling: blood begins to flow into the penis and it becomes warmer and thicker. Anything beyond level five is rigidity—that erection with a "spring back" quality. A level ten is an extremely hard erection, one that is almost painful.

You can easily achieve intercourse with an erection at about a level five. Based on this scale, most men have nothing to be concerned about. All of the sensate focus exercises in this book, whether they are for your partner alone or the two of you together, will help him have more satisfying erections, as they will teach him how to pay attention to what you are feeling. Peaking and plateauing will help him as well, as arousal is what fuels erections. You can also try the following techniques for better lovemaking.

♀ Exercise ♂
Daily Genital Massage

Every day, for ten minutes, gently massage your partner's penis, especially around the base. This is a way to get more blood flowing to the genital area. Put simply, this will help "prime the pump."

Don't caress or massage to create an erection. Massage for your partner to become aware of his penis and the sensations in it. This makes or reinforces the mind-body connection, which is crucial to experiencing deep arousal. Gentle massage will help develop his sensate focus awareness, in the same way as the earlier self-touch exercises in this book did.

Do this massage whether he has an erection or not. I promise you will see the results in future exercises.

♀ Exercise ♂
Erection Awareness

Sometimes men can get so out of touch with their own body that they do not know whether they have an erection or not. Basic sensate focus exercises such as the face, back, front, and genital caress will help your partner learn to experience sensations. If he does not have erection awareness, he may experience pleasant feelings while not being aware that his penis is hard enough for intercourse. I have worked with many clients who have this problem. It was common to have a session in which I would give a genital caress for twenty minutes or so and the client would have an erection almost the entire time without realizing it. Eventually the erection would go away simply because a lot of time had elapsed, and the client would think that in fact he had not had an erection at all.

Another cause of lack of erection awareness is that many men specifically learn to ignore their erections because they think that is the best way to get an erection. Actually this is partially on the right track. Men do need to stop worrying about their genitals and start feeling them. However, they want to concentrate on their genital sensations, not ignore them.

Before You Begin   To practice erection awareness, your partner should think of the hardness of his erection on the one-to-ten scale mentioned earlier. Remember that level one is a completely flaccid penis, level five is the beginning of rigidity, and level ten is an extremely hard, almost painful erection. If your partner has morning erections or erections when he masturbates, he should practice describing them using this scale.

The Exercise   For this first erection awareness exercise have your partner lie on his back. Begin a slow, focused front caress and genital caress for about twenty minutes. At various points ask him how strong he thinks his erection is. If your observation differs significantly from his estimate, ask him to open his eyes and look at his penis.

If he describes his erection as a two (beginning filling) when in fact it is a five (beginning rigidity, borderline hard) he needs to believe this. After he has seen his erection, he should close his eyes and concentrate on the feelings in his penis again as you continue your caress. This will help him learn to recognize the feelings of erection without having to look.

Remind your partner to keep his PC muscle and leg muscles relaxed, and to breathe and focus. Ask him about his erection level several more times. If you sense he's beginning to feel pressured to have an erection, back up to an earlier level of filling and slow down. There may not be that much variation in erections the first time you do the exercise. If you only hit erection levels of two or three, you have still made progress. Repeat the exercise as many times as you need to until he can reliably recognize some degree of rigidity.

Without a Partner   If your partner is uncomfortable doing this exercise with you, he can easily adapt it to do by himself. He simply does a genital caress, estimates hardness, then checks his sensations against perception.

♀ Exercise ♂
Getting and Losing Erections

This getting-and-losing exercise will help your partner develop a new, effective response for times when he feels his erection go down. What goes up must come down, but that's not such a bad thing, and it need not interrupt the flow of your lovemaking.

The Exercise   To begin the exercise, he lies on his back with his eyes closed. Begin a sensual front caress and a manual and oral genital caress. Whenever he gets a noticeable erection (even if it is only filling at levels two, three, and four), stop the stimulation and allow his erection to go all the way back down. Then start caressing again. If he gets another erection, stop. Each time during the caress let the erection get a little harder before stopping. Repeat this a number of times during a twenty-minute period.

The first time you do this exercise it may be frustrating. Your partner may not have an erection at all, because he is worrying about it. If he does have an erection, he may be tempted to fall back on old habits of flexing his PC muscle, tensing his thighs, thrusting his pelvis, or holding his breath when he feels himself losing the erection. Give him gentle feedback if he does this. You can help him monitor this so he becomes aware of the simple relationships: relaxation means blood flows in, tension means blood flows out.

Your partner may get frustrated the first few times you stop your strokes. He may think, "I'll show her! This time I'll get the erection and I won't lose it even though she stops stroking me." But he will—since this is the effect psychological pressure has.

Again, it is wonderful to be able to do this exercise together, but it is also very effective if he does it alone.

♀ Exercise ♂
Flaccid Insertion

Your partner may be having partial erections but avoiding using them for intercourse because he thinks they aren't hard enough. If he tends to put a lot of pressure on himself to have an erection, this exercise will illustrate the pleasures of intercourse without an erection. This technique is also wonderful if he has erection problems because of medical causes, and you desire the loving intimacy of intercourse.

The Exercise   Have him lie on his side facing you, as you lie on your back with one leg on top of his and the other in between. You will be at right angles to each other, with your genitals right up against each other.

Both of you should breathe and relax. Caress your genitals and his with lubricant. If he becomes partially erect during this, it is fine.

Regardless of his level of erection, gently fold or "stuff" his penis into your vagina. You can open your vagina with your fingers, and sometimes it is helpful to slide a flaccid penis into the vagina using one or two fingers as a splint. Rather than inserting the head of the penis first, you can also place the penis along the labia with the base at the vaginal opening. Then gently push the base of the penis into the vagina. The tip will naturally follow. Another way to insert a flaccid penis is to hold it tightly around the base between two of your fingers and push it into the vagina with your other hand.

Then, squeeze your PC muscle to make sure his penis is inside.

The purpose of this exercise is not for him to become aroused, but to experience being inside you with no pressure to have an erection or perform sexually. Once he is inside you, it may be tempting to move or thrust. The first time you do this exercise both of you should try to remain as still as possible. Breathe and relax your legs. At most, one of you can squeeze your PC muscle once in a while to make sure he is still inserted. Focus on non-pressured physical union with your lover.

Repeat this exercise adding a little more movement each time. Focus on the point of connection: your warmth, wetness, and the sexual energy. Eventually, allow your partner to peak up to different levels of arousal (not erection). If he focuses on what he is feeling and how aroused he is, he is more likely to get and maintain an erection.

♀ Exercise ♂
Oral Sex with the Man on Top

Does your partner have erections reliably but find it difficult to get one when he is lying on his back? If so, experiment with oral-genital caresses in a different position. Instead of having oral sex while he reclines, have him kneel on all fours while you lie perpendicular to him on your side. A pillow or two may make you more comfortable. From this position you can caress his penis and do pressure-free sensuous oral sex. It is a little more difficult for men to keep their legs relaxed when they are kneeling, but a lot of men find that in this position gravity gives them a little boost of blood flow.

More Fulfilling Erections

Here are some other points of mind-body connection that you both may want to consider in dealing with concerns about erections.

Attitude   The first place to start is with attitude and sexual awareness. Never pressure your partner to have an erection during any exercise. You can do any loving exercise in this book, up to and including intercourse, without an erection. While working through the exercises in this book, pay more attention to his arousal levels than to his erection. You will find that erections aren't the center of your ability to make love, they are part of it, an expression.

Health Habits   After examining attitudes, take a joint look at his health habits. Is he overweight? Does he smoke, drink alcohol, or use illegal drugs? All of these can cause erection problems. Quitting these

practices will make dramatic changes in his erections, sexual fulfillment, and ultimately, ability to make love.

Medical Conditions   Does he have any chronic medical conditions
that might be affecting his erections? Diabetes, prostate problems, and
circulation problems are among the medical conditions that can interfere with erections. In addition, many prescription medications, such
as those given for high blood pressure and ulcers, can affect erections.

Emotions   Lastly, look at your emotional landscape. Are either of you
depressed, anxious, or stressed out? Are you alienated from or unhappy
with each other? Is your relationship a mess? If it is, no wonder he
can't get an erection!

Pelvic Steal   In addition to all of the physical and emotional problems
that can affect erections, it is also possible that he may be doing some
things during lovemaking that prevent erections. Unconsciously or
consciously squeezing the PC muscle during stimulation can actually
prevent erection. As he becomes aroused he may also unconsciously
tighten the muscles in his legs, abdomen, or buttocks. Some men do
this because they think it helps them get an erection. In fact, it does
the opposite, because the blood that could be available for the erection is diverted to the muscles that are tightening up. This situation is
called pelvic steal syndrome: the blood that could be used for an erection is literally being stolen by the long muscles of the body.

Spectatoring   The term "spectatoring," coined by Masters and Johnson,
refers to watching and worrying about how you are doing in lovemaking. As they say, a watched pot never boils . . . and a watched penis
never hardens.

   If you have tried the exercises in this book and still feel that
there is a medical condition interfering with your partner's erection
process, and that his ability to make love will be enhanced by harder
erections, encourage him to consult a urologist who specializes in
medical treatments for erection problems.

Medical Aids for Erection

In the past, men who had erection problems due to medical conditions such as diabetes or prostate problems had few choices. They could opt to make love without an erection or they could opt for invasive surgery to place an implant in the penis. These implants came in two forms—a semi-rigid rod or an inflatable hydraulic device. Then a treatment for organic impotence was developed in which a muscle relaxant was injected directly into the erectile tissue of the penis. Many men found this unpleasant.

Today there are a number of treatments available for medically based erection problems. A man can insert a suppository (called MUSE) into the opening of the urethra, which will cause an erection in about ten minutes if he receives some stimulation. The most exciting new development in medical treatment for erection problems is Viagra (sildenafil). Viagra is taken orally, and if a man receives stimulation about one hour later he will get an erection. Another new development is being tested in which the medication is administered in wafer form and works in about twenty minutes. Because Viagra increases the action of nitric oxide, which helps smooth muscles relax, there is also some speculation about prescribing it for women who have difficulty becoming aroused. Initial studies of Viagra use in women have had positive results. Cautious optimism is warranted, as side effects include nausea and vision changes.

Inhibited Ejaculation

This problem was once called "ejaculatory incompetence" or "retarded ejaculation." This was quite confusing, because orgasm and ejaculation are not the same thing. Orgasm is a delicious, full-body experience: it makes your heart pound, speeds up breathing, sends spasms through the long muscles in your arms and legs, and ends with an intense feeling of release. The energy built up in your body heightens to a peak and is released rapidly. Some people feel an altered state of consciousness during orgasm.

Ejaculation, on the other hand, is a physiological act—the release of semen propelled by PC muscle spasms. A man can have an orgasm without ejaculating. He can also have an ejaculation without an orgasm or without even feeling good. It is also possible for men to have multiple orgasms the same way women can, as you know from reading Chapter 9.

Most men and women in this culture expect a man to have an ejaculation (accompanied by an orgasm) every time he has intercourse. But all men are different, and there are many men who have difficulty ejaculating during intercourse and are concerned about it. This difficulty with ejaculation may stem from masturbation habits or chronic PC muscle tension.

If your partner has difficulty ejaculating during intercourse, and if this causes him concerns that interfere with his ability to express his love to you, try the following exercises. The PC muscle exercises will help him learn to relax his PC muscle as he becomes very aroused. The bonding exercises will help you both feel closer, and the peaking and plateauing exercises will make him more aware of his arousal levels so that he doesn't anticipate ejaculation too soon.

♀ Exercise ♂
Softening the Stroke

Here is a special set of exercises to help your partner sensitize his penis. They will help him become more aware of the delicate sensations of being inside your vagina.

One of the most common causes of difficulty with ejaculation is a man's masturbation style. If his stroke is too fast or he applies too much pressure, it desensitizes his penis. If your partner used to or still does masturbate frequently (once a day or more), he should try cutting back in order to give his penis time to re-sensitize. He can also try limiting his masturbation time to ten or fifteen minutes to retrain himself to ejaculate more quickly. He may also find, during this process, that different strokes can bring him to climax.

The following exercise is one for your partner to do alone, when masturbating. Alternatively, you might suggest doing this together, with you providing the stroking.

The Exercise (For Men Alone) Do a genital caress, with eyes closed, and concentrate on the sensations of your touch. As you caress, slow down your stroke so that it is half as fast as when you began. Enjoy the sensations of this new stroke. What changes do you feel in your penis, your fingers?

Now slow down a second time, until your fingers and palm are barely moving over your penis. Continue this caress for fifteen minutes, whether you ejaculate or not.

Use this exercise on a regular basis to decrease your masturbation frequency, time, and the roughness of your stroke. To help slow yourself down, you can try using your left hand if you are right-handed (or vice versa), or using an open palm or fingertips instead of using a closed fist.

♀ Exercise ♂
Alternating Peaks

This exercise is especially enjoyable because it encourages your partner to savor the unique touches of both oral stimulation and intercourse.

The Exercise Begin a peaking exercise in which you do a genital caress on your partner up through a strong level. He should focus on the sensations and texture of your touch. Then begin intercourse and peak up again. Really feel the sensations of your mutual touch.

Next, give your partner an oral genital caress until he peaks to an urgent level. Let him really experience the different touches of your tongue and lips. Return to having intercourse until he reaches the next peak.

Continue alternating oral caress peaks with intercourse peaks. Repeat the exercise until he is able to ejaculate with an intercourse peak.

As a variation on this exercise you might also wish to alternate peaks in which he stimulates himself.

♀ Exercise ♂
Approaching Intercourse

This is another approach to inhibited ejaculation that I have seen work with many men. Do a peaking exercise with your partner in which he peaks himself up to an urgent level of arousal. When he feels he is on the verge of ejaculating, insert his penis into your vagina.

Repeat this exercise so he can enjoy the feeling of ejaculation in addition to the feeling of being inside you. He can try entering just before "the point of no return" until he can enter you at a less urgent level and build to ejaculation.

● ● ●

When you have difficulty ejaculating, it's easy to get caught up in a performance mode. Try not to forget the sensate focus principles and the loving mindset as you do these exercises. Also, women often tend to have a better sense than men of how to make love without performance pressure. Your attitude can often affect your partner positively in this way.

Chapter 12
Loving Women

Women also have sexual concerns or problems that can interfere with making love. This chapter covers making love with a woman who has such sexual concerns or problems, just as the last chapter covered making love with a man who has sexual concerns or problems. As I said in the last chapter, it is important that women and men understand and support each other if they have sexual concerns. Partners can do a lot to help each other, and for that reason most of this chapter about women is written for their male partner, just as most of the previous chapter about men was addressed to their female partner.

The information in this chapter covers the most common concerns that women have about their sexuality. It also includes specific single and couple exercises that will allow you to actually treat a problem together by making love in the sensate focus manner. Because women are more likely than men to have experienced sexual abuse or trauma, which can lead to an inability to make love, some of the exercises in this chapter are for women to do on their own, with whatever degree of support or involvement they want from their partner.

The most common female sexual concerns are female sexual arousal disorder, low or no arousal, trouble achieving orgasms, and sexual pain problems of vaginismus and dyspareunia.

Women's Sexual Arousal

When women become sexually aroused, there are both physical and psychological changes that take place. As a woman is aroused physically, her clitoris, outer lips, inner lips, and vaginal tissues swell as blood fills them. Most women also experience some degree of vaginal lubrication. This is caused when the blood flow into the vaginal walls pushes moisture into the vagina. However, most women who complain of arousal difficulties complain that they do not feel aroused psychologically, that they don't feel themselves swelling up or lubricating.

Does your partner have difficulty becoming aroused? Is she aware of her arousal sensations? Many women aren't. Arousal problems can be caused by a number of factors, and one of these is that women often don't recognize the physical signs of arousal.

Some women become concerned because they don't lubricate adequately or often. I have found that lubrication is not a reliable sign of psychological or emotional arousal. The amount of a woman's lubrication can fluctuate with hormonal levels and age. Your partner might lubricate without feeling turned on at all; conversely, she could be very turned on but not lubricate. Some women notice that the decrease in estrogen after menopause causes their vaginal tissues to become dry. You are better off using the arousal awareness scale as an indication rather than the wetness between her legs. If your partner does have difficulty lubricating, however, be sure to use an artificial lubricant so she stays comfortable.

Many exercises in the earlier sections of this book, especially the arousal awareness, peaking, and plateauing exercises, are helpful in allowing women to experience increased arousal. If, after those exercises, your partner still continues to experience difficulty becoming aroused, the first thing to try is simply slowing down and savoring your mutual sexual explorations. This has helped many women: to slow down and enjoy more genital caressing and oral sex from their partner before beginning intercourse. Having you penetrate too soon can either cause arousal problems for your partner or make them worse. So can passively accepting whatever stimulation you want to give her. So, a second solution for low arousal is for your partner to become more active. You may both receive a psychological boost from her being in charge.

♀ Exercise ♂
Getting Active for Arousal

In this exercise you remain passive throughout. Lie on your back, close your eyes, and try not to move. Your partner will pretend your body is a playground or a toy for her to play with. She can play with you, stroke, caress, lick, or suck on your body. Whatever she decides to do, she should do it slowly, sensuously, and without any pressure on either of you. If she wants to climb on top of you and have intercourse, she should. Chances are that at some point in this exercise you won't be able to hold still any longer, and the two of you can revel in your sexual play together.

Exercise for Women Alone
Exploring Your Vagina

Here is a great exercise for women to do alone. It will help a woman discover her unique pleasure spots and explore the depths of her arousal potential, and can help her work through issues of pain on penetration in a way that feels safe.

Probably the most common cause of a woman's difficulty in becoming aroused is not knowing her own body. The self-touch exercises in Chapters 3 and 4 will help you a lot with that. Here is a more advanced exercise that will allow you to explore your vagina.

Before You Begin   Buy a dildo that is about the same size and shape as your partner's penis. (See the next section.)

The Exercise   Lie comfortably on a bed and have the dildo ready to use. Breathe deeply and relax. Begin to give yourself a slow, languid genital caress. Use plenty of lubricant. Slowly insert a finger about one knuckle's length into your vagina. Practice squeezing and relaxing your PC muscle around your finger, till you are comfortable inserting it all the way into your vagina.

Put some lubricant on the dildo and slowly, sensuously stroke your clitoris, outer lips, and inner lips with it. Now insert it and rub it along the front wall of your vagina about two inches in. Can you feel your G spot? It will feel very sensitive and putting pressure on it may make you feel that you want to urinate. Gradually move the dildo into your vagina as deep as it will go. Bring your legs up and back if this helps you insert the dildo. Remember to stay focused and to breathe and relax. Can you feel your cervix? It will feel like a hard lump toward the back of your vagina. Some women find stimulation of the cervix very arousing. Do you?

Experiment with running the dildo up and down your vaginal walls. See if there are any areas that you find particularly sensitive. The vagina has many more areas that can trigger stimulation than experts previously thought.

If you feel yourself becoming very aroused during this exercise, do a couple of high-level peaks. Then stimulate yourself to orgasm if you wish.

A Note on Buying Sexual Aids

If you have never used a dildo or vibrator, you probably have some resistance to the idea. You may even feel a little shy about purchasing one. My sincere recommendation is to go ahead and get it. Using a penis-shaped object is the best and most stimulating way I know of to promote a woman's arousal and orgasms. At the end of this chapter I have listed the names of some companies I have dealt with that sell both penis-shaped and non–penis-shaped sexual aids, and sell them discreetly.

If the idea of a buying or using a penis-shaped object makes you uncomfortable, for any reason, look through a catalog and select a non–penis-shaped one that feels right.

Orgasms Come in All Colors, Shapes, and Sizes

One of the most common sexual problems that women have is difficulty having an orgasm (especially during intercourse). This can definitely interfere with a woman's ability to give love freely during a sexual encounter.

Many women don't know what happens during orgasm. Though this is less likely to be true for someone over forty, if your partner has not been very orgasmic or comes from a background where she didn't get a chance to discuss sexual matters, she may not know what feelings to expect, and may not recognize her orgasm for what it is.

When a woman has an orgasm, the muscles around her uterus and cervix will spasm, so that her abdomen flutters. She may expel some air from her vagina. Blood flows into the vaginal walls, creating pressure that causes a flow of lubrication. Blood pressure, heart rate, and breathing all reach a peak. Her neck, arm, face, and leg muscles may spasm involuntarily, and tension in her PC muscle causes it to spasm shortly after. She may feel a tingling sensation in some parts of her body and a sensation of warmth that begins in her pelvis and spreads through to her chest, neck, and face. And the skin of her face, neck, and chest may flush. For more information, consult my book *Super Sexual Orgasm.*

During orgasm, the sympathetic nervous system and parasympathetic nervous system both work at the same time. Sexual energy builds up and is released rapidly, leading to a state of relief, euphoria, and sometimes even to altered consciousness. Some women have "gushers" with their orgasms—female ejaculations, in which fluid is expelled from the vagina. You may have heard that gushers are a myth, but they are real. They occur with intense stimulation of the G spot, the extremely sensitive area in the upper front wall of the vagina.

This all sounds positively earth shattering, doesn't it? But the reality for most women is that orgasms vary in intensity. Sometimes a woman may experience voluptuous, full-body orgasms and at other times she might feel simple PC quivers and a mildly pleasant sensation of release. If she weren't paying attention, she might even miss it.

Over the years, women have put incredible amounts of pressure on themselves to have orgasms. Some women make the mistake of expecting every orgasm to be a major one and are disappointed if they have a mild orgasm. Lots of women expect too much from orgasm, and make it into a goal of life-changing proportions. Becoming orgasmic will and won't change your partner's life: her lovemaking will be more euphoric, her body will feel better, and her health will improve. But as far as I can tell, orgasm won't make her richer or thinner, make your kids behave, or keep the house clean. I encourage all women not to pressure themselves to have orgasms. What is important is that women open themselves to their orgasmic capacity in whatever ways feel good to them.

As with desire, the type of stimulation that leads to orgasm and the delights of the orgasm itself are unique for every woman. Women need to get comfortable with their individual levels and patterns of orgasm, and learn to accept them. Over time this frees them to enjoy and deepen that response.

Increasing Orgasms

Though some women have never *felt* an orgasm, I believe that just about every woman has *had* an orgasm at some time in her life. She may have had one as a child, or in a dream or fantasy, but may not have recognized her feelings and her release as orgasmic. More important, my experience is that every woman can be orgasmic. An orgasm is a basic body reflex, like yawning or sneezing, which is prompted by a satisfactory level of arousal. The key is for a woman to discover her individual orgasmic pathway.

Some women strive for orgasm during intercourse not so much because it feels good, but because they wish to share this loving expression of intense arousal, vulnerability, and abandon with their partner. You two will find through the following exercises that orgasm can heighten her senses and deepen your intimate connection.

The first step for your partner to develop her orgasmic potential is to explore her body and learn about her sexual responses. Lack of knowledge about her individual response is the single biggest cause of a woman's inability to have orgasms. She cannot depend on you to always know what excites her, though the exercises in Chapters 3 and 5 will deepen her self-knowledge and the partner exercises in Chapter 6 will help you. Chances are, if your partner is healthy, these basics of sexual loving will take her to the brink of orgasm and beyond. In fact, you may not need anything else. However, if you do go all the way through this program and your partner is still not orgasmic, but would like to be, here are some secrets. . . .

Exercise for Women Alone
Masturbating with a Dildo

A woman's key to arousal and eventual orgasm during intercourse is realizing the importance of the PC muscle spasms. Unless your PC muscle is in great shape, it is hard for it to spasm when you have something (anything) in your vagina. To practice becoming more orgasmic during intercourse, practice with the dildo you bought for the previous exercise.

The Exercise Give yourself a slow genital caress with the dildo. Keep the touch sensual, and remember to breathe and focus on your sensations. Insert the dildo, tease your PC muscle with it, and begin to peak. Squeeze and relax your PC muscle around the dildo, and caress your clitoris. Explore what feels good. When you reach the point of orgasm, insert the dildo just as your PC muscle starts to spasm.

♀ Exercise ♂
Masturbating with Your Partner's Penis

This is a sexy exercise to increase your partner's sexual self-awareness and encourage her to act on her own desires (but I guarantee it is enjoyable for both parties involved!).

The Exercise Exchange sensual genital caresses and oral sex until you have a strong erection and your partner is quite aroused. Your partner then lies on her back with her legs up, and you kneel between her legs. Caress the opening of her vagina with your penis. Slowly tease her PC muscle by inserting only an inch and then withdrawing.

At all times, let her ask for and control what you do. She might ask you to alternate caressing her clitoris and stroking her PC muscle with your penis. After a few minutes of this, she could have you insert all the way and thrust deeply a few times. If her PC muscle is tuned up from previous exercises, it will begin to quiver and flutter around your penis and may bring her to orgasmic spasms. Remember, you move, caress, and thrust exactly as she asks you to, while she focuses on her own arousal as it builds up and releases.

♀ Exercise ♂
Orgasm on Impact

Many women think that the more time they spend in intercourse, the more likely they are to have an orgasm. Not surprisingly, a lot of men think this too. It is a myth. The truth is, if you are aroused enough during intercourse to have an orgasm, it will usually occur within about seven minutes. The next exercise shows your partner that she doesn't need to spend extended amounts of time having intercourse in order to orgasm. She can learn to come within one or two strokes of penetration. The real secret to this exercise is in practicing peaking, not in the penetration itself.

The Exercise Let your partner begin by giving you a sensuous oral caress. When you become erect, she climbs astride you and slowly stimulates herself by rubbing her clitoris and vaginal lips against your penis, but doesn't insert it. In this way she peaks a couple of times at strong levels of arousal.

In between her peaks, she can have oral sex with you so you maintain a high arousal level.

Your partner should peak to an urgent arousal level by slowly rubbing your penis on her clitoris and outside her vagina. While she does, keep your leg muscles and PC muscle as relaxed as possible. She should keep her eyes closed and speed up her breathing. When she comes to the brink of orgasm, she opens her eyes, takes a deep breath, and thrusts herself all the way down upon you. She will likely reach orgasm within about five strokes.

Enjoy practicing this exercise until your partner can have an orgasm on the first stroke. If she peaks herself to a very urgent level of arousal several times before penetration, rather than just once or twice, it increases her likelihood of having an immediate orgasm.

♀ Exercise ♂
Orgasm on Impact (Using the PC Muscle)

Your partner can also use her PC muscle to help her orgasm on your first stroke. Do the exercise as described above, but when she sits on your penis, in addition to opening her eyes and taking a deep breath, she slams her PC muscle shut around the shaft of your penis. This will often trigger a powerful orgasm, especially if her PC muscle is already fluttering on the edge.

♀ Exercise ♂
The Bridge to Orgasm

Although this sounds like something out of engineering school, it's actually a gratifying way to bring your partner's self-discovery together with your sexual partnership. This technique creates a psychological, behavioral bridge between her ability to orgasm when stimulating her clitoris and her ability to orgasm with intercourse.

The Exercise Lie on your back as your partner does a front caress and genital caress to arouse you. When you become erect, she will climb on top of you and begin peaking and plateauing, using your penis to pleasure herself. As she reaches strong and then urgent peaks and plateaus, she stimulates her clitoris with her fingers, and masturbates to orgasm while your penis strokes her. With some practice she will need less and less direct clitoral stimulation with her fingers, and her ability to have an orgasm will transfer to the stimulation of intercourse.

There are two variations of this exercise. Both work best if she is on top. You can stimulate her clitoris with your hand instead of her doing it herself. Or, either one of you can use a vibrator or dildo to stimulate her. She can also practice alternating peaks with the dildo, your hand, her hand, and your penis.

♀ Exercise ♂
Fake It till You Make It

Here is a very intense exercise to try if your partner is still having difficulty reaching orgasm. "Imitating orgasm" is not faking an orgasm to please you, to make you think she's having one when she's not. Instead, by imitating orgasm, she learns to fake her body into thinking she is having an orgasm—which often triggers a real orgasm. This is most likely to help if she can peak up to a very urgent level of arousal but can't seem to go over the edge.

The Exercise   The orgasmic response is a full body response, not something that occurs only in the genitals. At the moment of orgasm, your face contorts, your arms, neck, and legs spasm, and your PC muscle begins to contract. If your partner enacts these body responses when she is at an urgent arousal level, there is a good chance that she can trigger an orgasm.

When you are making love and your partner reaches the height of her arousal, have her take a deep breath, suck in her lower abdomen, hunch her shoulders into the bed, thrust her pelvis up, open her eyes wide, and relax her PC muscle. This may trigger a real orgasm, which she will experience as a fluttering or spasming of the PC muscle.

Another way for her to do this is to wait until she is on the brink of orgasm and then slam her PC muscle shut instead of relaxing it. This can often trigger the necessary spasms.

A third alternative is for her to pretend she is having an orgasm and to act the way she thinks highly orgasmic women act. Pretending that she is highly arousable and orgasmic may allow you both to practice orgasm techniques in a nonthreatening way, until she feels more comfortable with them.

All of these methods of triggering orgasm have several things in common. First, your partner learns to focus, breathe, and relax enough to allow herself to climb to exquisite, intense arousal. She learns to focus enough to avoid having any distracting thoughts when she reaches climactic levels of arousal.

These orgasm techniques are not ends in themselves but are ways for your partner to accustom herself to having orgasms. As she becomes familiar with the power of these triggers, she will be able to use them with intercourse. As with any skill that involves learning complex patterns of behavior and combining them, the first few tries may feel artificial. After she practices these techniques for a while, they become automatic and her relaxation and arousal levels will lead her to fulfilling orgasms.

Vaginismus

Vaginismus is a very frustrating condition in which a woman's PC muscle, which also surrounds the opening of the vagina, goes into a painful, uncontrolled spasm. As a result, the vagina tightens up and the woman's partner cannot enter her. Vaginismus can be caused by anxiety, lack of sexual knowledge, sexual trauma, or abuse.

If your partner has vaginismus, spend lots of time with the bonding exercises in Chapter 2, and encourage her to do the self-touch exercises in Chapters 3 and 5. If you are not able to insert a finger in her vagina during the genital caress don't worry, just caress the outside. Then do the partner exercises in Chapter 6, up to the genital caress. At that point, your partner can spend time alone doing the solo exercises for vaginal pain given below. When she is ready, the two of you can explore the gentle couple exercises also included in this section.

Exercise for Women Alone
Finger Penetration for Vaginismus

This is a special exercise for you to try when you reach the stage where you can do the genital caress with some finger penetration by yourself. Slowly caress your clitoris and vaginal lips using sensate focus techniques. Breathe and relax. Relax your PC muscle and try to insert the tip of your little finger into your vagina just one-half inch. Tighten your PC muscle around your fingertip and then relax it. Now see if you can insert it an inch. Tighten, and relax again. Keep going with this until you can insert each finger on each hand one at a time all the way in. If at any time you feel pain, don't push yourself, but back up to a stage you feel comfortable with.

♀ Exercise ♂
Penetration with Loving Fingers

This exercise brings your loving energy to your partner's explorations. Lie down in a comfortable position and have your partner lie next to you. After she caresses herself with her hand and fingers, she takes your hand and gradually inserts each of your fingers, from the smallest to the largest, into her vagina one at a time, tightening and relaxing her PC muscle at each stage. You should use plenty of lubrication. Keep your hand totally relaxed and don't become active in any way, because the important thing is that she is in charge of the depth and timing of any penetration.

Exercise for Women Alone
Penetration with a Dildo

Buy a dildo that appeals to you and is about halfway between the size of a finger and your partner's penis. Make yourself comfortable, and then follow the steps of the penetration exercise above using the dildo instead of your partner's fingers. Remember to breathe, relax, and focus on positive, sensual, loving feelings.

♀ Exercise ♂
Penetration with Your Flaccid Penis

Follow the exercise for flaccid insertion in Chapter 11, but have your partner insert your penis one-half inch at a time instead of all at once. Then progress to doing this exercise with your partially erect penis and, eventually, with a full erection. After she is comfortable inserting you when you are fully erect, try the exercise in positions other than side-to-side. If you find yourself becoming too erect, use your breathing or tighten your hip and thigh muscles to soften your erection. The important thing is that she stays in charge of the timing, depth, and angle of penetration until she is comfortable having you do it. At that point, you will be ready to try some of the advanced intercourse exercises from Chapter 7.

Dyspareunia

Dyspareunia is pain during intercourse that has psychological causes. If your partner experiences pain during intercourse, she should first rule out all possible physical causes, which may include menstrual problems, tumors, ovarian cysts, venereal disease, pelvic infections, endometriosis, or an injury such as a pulled muscle or torn ligament.

It is unlikely that a physical abnormality of the vagina is causing her problem.

If she has been to a physician and ruled out physical causes, it is likely that her pain during intercourse has a psychological origin. This is especially likely if she experiences sharp, piercing vaginal pain during intercourse, since the vagina does not actually have the nerve endings to feel that type of pain.

The first step to healing dyspareunia so that you and your partner can fully express sexual love is for your partner to get comfortable with the basic exercises that are recommended for everybody, such as self-touch, bonding, and partner exercises. When doing caresses, particularly genital caresses, don't continue anything that causes her pain. Look for her physical cues, such as tensing or wincing, as well as verbal ones. After you have begun to develop momentum with the bonding and partner exercises, try the following.

Exercise for Women Alone
Exploring Your Vagina (for Sexual Pain)

During a genital caress, insert your finger into your vagina as far as is comfortable. When you reach a point where you feel pain, back off and only do the caress up to the point where the pain starts. (Remember, if you cannot insert a finger at all, you have vaginismus, not dyspareunia).

The next time you do this exercise, use a small dildo instead of your finger. Insert the dildo to the point where you are afraid you might feel pain. Relax your PC muscle and see if you can insert the dildo a little farther. Remember to breathe slowly and deeply, and keep your legs and all other muscles relaxed. Make a mark on the dildo to show how far you inserted it. Each time you repeat the exercise, see if you can insert the dildo a little farther without pain. Your goal is to become comfortable with penetration, so you can penetrate without pain.

♀ Exercise ♂
Penetration with Your Penis (for Sexual Pain)

Lie on your back as your partner stimulates you with sensuous caresses until you have an erection. Then caress plenty of lubrication onto her genital area, while she climbs on top and slowly inserts your penis a half-inch at a time. If she reaches a point where she feels pain, she should stop. Remind her to breathe and relax her PC muscle. She can slowly thrust all the way up and down on your penis as long as it doesn't hurt her. She should stay in control of all the thrusting—you simply lie passively, without moving.

Repeat intercourse in this way until she is comfortable enough for you to start moving. You can begin by slightly, sensuously rolling your hips. When that becomes comfortable for her, try changing positions and exploring some of the more advanced intercourse exercises in Chapter 7.

If this exercise is difficult for your partner, or she doesn't feel ready for it, she should do the previous solo exercise, "Exploring Your Vagina (for Sexual Pain)," a few times first.

If your partner has difficulty becoming aroused or being orgasmic, or if she has severe vaginismus or sexual pain, her problems may be due to trauma or abuse in her past. If that is the case, encourage her to consult a qualified therapist who can help her deal with these problems.

• • •

As a man, there is a lot you can share with your partner about enjoying making love—men and women traditionally have different sexual strengths. Women can teach men to be less performance-oriented. Men can share with women their sexual enthusiasm and good-old-fashioned horniness. The more you as a man can connect with that feeling of sexual vigor and energy you felt as a young man, the more you will be able to infect your partner with your enthusiasm.

Mail Order Sources

The companies below sell dildos, vibrators, and other sexual aids through the mail. While I am not endorsing any of these companies, they all have excellent reputations.

Good Vibrations
San Francisco, CA
1-415-974-8990
(call for catalog)

Intimate Treasures
San Francisco, CA
1-415-863-5002
(call for catalog)

Xandria Collection
Department C 1096
P.O. Box 31039
San Francisco, CA 94131-9988
(write for catalog)

Lady Calston
908 Niagara Falls Blvd., Suite 519
North Tonawanda, NY 14120-2060
1-800-690-5239

Adam and Eve
P.O. Box 900
Department CS 357
Carrboro, NC 27510
1-800-274-0333

Chapter 13
The Loving Spirit

A s we get older, we often begin to look for more meaning in what we do and experience, and to look for the universal in the particular. Habits or peculiarities that annoyed us about a partner not too long ago now somehow become endearing evidence of how human he or she is, how fallible we all are, how easily we fool ourselves into thinking we're fooling everyone else. In undertaking the journey of making love better than ever we moved from having just passion and arousal in our relationship, or just compatibility and liking, to wanting it all working together, an intimate, lustful, sexually regenerative companionship. Now we come to the revelation—and it *is* that—that making love in a committed and passionate relationship can connect both of you with something larger than either of you.

I don't consider myself particularly religious or spiritual, but I do know that you are missing something in life if you don't have a feeling for the transpersonal, even if the connection you feel is simply with nature. I have saved this discussion until last because it is not so much a conclusion as a jumping off point, an introduction to another vista of your relationship—sacred sexuality. While some of you may relate to it, others may not.

The path to sacred sexuality is one you have already embarked on. Getting in touch with the physical aspects of sexual expression is the beginning. The next step, which I hope this book helps you take, is using the sensate focus exercises and the loving mindset to add mutuality, intimacy, and commitment. Now you have an opportunity to infuse the partnership you have built with mindfulness, loving intention, and a sense of the unity that embraces us all. And from there, you may glimpse the transcendent.

Perhaps you have already experienced the transpersonal or transcendental element of lovemaking. Have you ever felt an altered state of consciousness, in which everything looked clearer or brighter after uniquely passionate sex? Scientifically, we can explain this euphoric state as the result of hyperventilation and endorphin release, but that shortchanges the profound effects such sexual connection can have on us. Many couples find that sexual union is a way to realize their connection with a higher power, whether they feel that power is God or the goddess, nature or goodness.

It's not as big a leap as you might think—just look at the sexuality occurring all around you! If you think about it, nature is nothing but sexual expression: seeds are sown, flowers bloom, bees carry pollen back to the hive in order to take part in a complex mating dance. Once we realize this, we begin to see how natural it is for us as humans to seek and thrive from sexual relationships. Understanding the naturalness of sexual expression can prepare us for the profound release and mystical connections it can bring.

Sexuality is also intimately connected to creativity, fertility, and exploration. We need to get comfortable with these aspects of universal and personal sexuality if we want to share in the loving spirit. We need to make a divine space for our partners and ourselves—whether through cultural traditions, personal rituals, creative expressions, or celebrations.

World Traditions of Sacred Sexuality

Throughout time, cultural traditions have recognized the power of lovemaking, often tying it into their cosmology, or theory of the universe. The Taoist tradition is based on the celebration of the Five Senses. The Bible includes "The Song of Songs," a lavish and beautiful poem that celebrates lovemaking. Hindu tradition includes a focus on how sexual energy both created and is a way to transcend this world. The teachings of the Jewish Kabbalah contain many erotic passages. The Islamic religion includes erotic love poetry. And on, and on.

For some people, the idea that religion contains a tradition of sacred sex is very threatening. So many of us have been brought up in a puritanical culture that suppresses sexuality rather than celebrating it. In direct conflict with this, our popular culture commercializes sexuality. As a result, many of us have learned to avoid sex, or isolate or fetishize it in our lifestyle, because our conflicted religious and cultural backgrounds insist that we associate the body and its sexual impulses with either shame and guilt or seduction and exploitation. What we really need is to integrate and embrace our sexuality, just as we embrace our partners.

♀ Exercise ♂
Studying the Sexual Spirit

Understanding the historical role of sexuality in your religious tradition can help heal the disjunction you might feel between spirituality and sexuality. Sexual loving can make it possible to resolve these attitudes and allow your sexual relationship to enrich you spiritually as well as physically and emotionally.

Sexuality permeates many traditions noted for sexual aspects. These are not so much religious traditions as cultural traditions, enriched by history, each generation's interpretation, and each individual personal experience. Whatever your religious background, you may find it helpful to understand what other cultures have passed on about sacred sexuality. Spend one or two nights at the library or at a bookstore, and read a sampling of the *Kama Sutra* or *The Perfumed Garden*. Then, if you are a member of an organized religion, find out what your religious tradition has to say about lovemaking as an expression of your spirituality and your relationship with the deity.

Let the richness of these traditions inform your own relationship with your sexuality and your spirituality. Share your discoveries with your partner, and discuss how you both feel about these traditions.

If you and your partner enjoy poetry, you may like to read selections of sacred sexual verse to each other in the evenings, or during quiet or romantic times that you set aside.

♀ Exercise ♂
The Cherishing Foot Bath

This exercise is not only sensual, it is also symbolic of humility and service. You may do this clothed or in the nude, whichever way you and your partner feel most comfortable and close.

Before You Begin You will need two towels, body soap, and lotion, and a basin filled with hot water, large enough for a person's feet.

The Exercise To begin, the person being bathed reclines in a chair, feet resting on the floor. The washer fills the basin with warm water, gently places the bather's feet in the water, and begins to gently wash and tend to them.

The foot bath is like any other sensate focus exercise: Use a light, caressing touch, rather than a massage. Bathe one foot at a time, finding out how the different areas of the foot feel as you bathe them. Stroke the ankles, the arches, and the tender underside of the toes. Focus on tending to your partner's feet with loving care. Although you touch for your own pleasure, believe me, your partner will like this one!

When you are finished, gently lift your partner's feet from the basin one at a time, pat them dry, and wrap them in separate towels. Put aside the basin, then take one foot from the towel, warm up some lotion in your palms and caress the foot with lotion.

When you are the person being bathed, relax and enjoy yourself. Feel what it is like to be cared for and tended to. Give yourself over to the ministrations or your partner. Allow yourself to be pampered.

♀ Exercise ♂
The Five Senses

Spend an afternoon or evening nurturing your partner's full spirit by engaging all five of the senses in lovemaking. Find symbols of earth, air, fire, and water, the four elements. What you bring to this ritual is the fifth element: your spirit.

In private, prepare a room for lovemaking with things that will feed the five senses: sight, smell, sound, taste, and touch. You may want to choose them around a theme. For example, if it is June, you can celebrate the current season by setting out a bowl of fragrant citrus blossoms (to appeal to your partner's sense of smell), opening the curtains to the summer skies or the summer moon (appealing to sight), and hanging windchimes that might chime in the summer breeze (sound). You can serve summer fruit such as watermelon, pomegranate, or pineapple to stimulate the taste buds, and use tanning oil to massage or caress your partner as a gift of touch. Be careful not to have too many things going on. One stimulus for each sense is enough.

On another night, your partner can be the bearer of delights for you. When you are receiving the five elements your partner has prepared for you, try to empty yourself of thoughts and open yourself to your senses. Focus on each sense, one at a time, and then experience them as a whole. Then experience them with your partner.

This exercise allows you to combine sensate focus with the sensual pleasures you know your partner likes, and also make a symbolic and real connection between lovemaking with your partner and the outward symbols of spiritual and cultural traditions, such as candles and wine.

♀ Exercise ♂
Fertility (or Creativity) Dinner

The breaking of bread and the sharing of food can be a symbolic ceremony. For example, the Jewish tradition of Passover commemorates the Jews' flight out of Egypt and each food served at a Passover supper holds symbolic meaning.

Have you and your partner gone through difficult times? Are you two trying to reach a new stage in your lives or your relationship? Do you cherish special aspects of your relationship? Share a symbolic fertility dinner to cultivate that energy and set the stage for your future together.

Consider this dinner a ritual or ceremony. Plan it in advance, with thought, so that it has a structure and meaning for the two of you. Serve special foods that symbolize fertility and creativity, such as fruits, flowers, and grains. Present the food in a beautiful manner, whether as a buffet or in separate courses. You may want to write or read poetry or other passages that celebrate fertility, rejuvenation, or the cycles of nature. Or, you may take the opportunity to discuss the ideas and ideals you hope to bring to fruition together.

♀ Exercise ♂
Personal Altars

Practitioners of some eastern religions often keep altars in their homes. They light candles or incense and meditate and pray before their altar. Some Christians do this also. In a similar way, you can create an altar to honor your relationship.

Make a space in your bedroom or another private room in your house, and build a shrine to your relationship. Together, select pictures of each other and the family or things you've created together. You might include historical objects, such as a first gift, or mementos of trips you've taken together, such as a stone or a seashell. Perhaps there are things that mark the stages of your life together—a college pennant, a matchbox from dinner out on a special anniversary, the calendar page that commemorates your first date. You might also include universal symbols such as mandalas (symbols of the universe), spirals (symbols of an inner journey), or suns (symbols of life), artwork that symbolizes male and female fertility, and things that represent your goals for the future. You can scent your altar with incense, dried flowers, or essential oils.

Once you have built your altar, tend to it. Rearrange the pictures, hold or finger the mementos and symbols. Let the experiences of your past and present come together with your hopes and aspirations for the future.

Tantra

The religious or sacred tradition that has the most to say about lovemaking is tantra—a form of yoga done in couples that comes from

India. The tantric cosmology features a whole theory of the universe created by male and female forces. The universe springs from the union of the god Shiva (pure consciousness) and his consort Shakti (pure energy). The difference between most forms of yoga that you may be familiar with and tantra is that most yoga preaches asceticism—getting away from the worldly and the material—whereas tantra teaches how to reach toward the sublime through ultra-sensual experience, becoming material, corporal, and earthy, while seeing and acknowledging the divine in the material. The most profound way to do this is by making love.

In tantra, the man and woman making love symbolize the male and female forces that created and power the universe. The male and female genitals are revered objects of worship. Tantra includes exercises, positions, rituals, and sexual postures that all have meaning in the tantric belief system. I hosted a *Playboy* video called "A Guide to Tantric Lovemaking" that shows modern couples how to do some of these exercises and practices, a few of which are quite weird by Western standards. For example, one of the tantric practices is to have sex for twenty-four hours straight during a full moon with a woman who is having her period, and another is for a man to make love for many hours and withhold ejaculation. But some of the sexual practices that have tantric roots are very erotic and can help you appreciate the part of your relationship that is sacred.

If you would like to explore tantra, I recommend beginning with the Playboy video or reading an introduction to tantra. Three excellent books on this art are *The Art of Sexual Ecstasy* and *The Art of Sexual Magic* by Margo Anand, and *Sexual Energy Ecstasy* by David and Ellen Ramsdale. There are also a number of workshops for those who would like specific training in tantra; you can usually find these by checking in the classifieds section of free weekly papers, or magazines such as *New Age Journal*.

Here is an exercise to introduce you to the energies from which tantra draws its power.

♀ Exercise ♂
Chakra Massage

The chakras are centers or vortices where various types of energies—physical, emotional, mental, and electromagnetic—are exchanged or connected with the world around us. Traditionally, there are seven chakras, which run along the spine and up to the head, reflecting the development of human consciousness. These chakras are located at the base of the spine (the "root center"), pelvis, navel or solar plexus, heart, throat, forehead (or "third eye"), and the crown of the head.

To release energy from these centers, do sensate focus caresses that start at the head chakras and move down to the pelvis to concentrate energy there. Concentrate on getting in touch with and feeling this energy. You can do a sensate focus exercise in which you caress only one chakra at a time for fifteen or twenty minutes. For example, you and your partner might want to take turns caressing each other's forehead.

Or, as an alternative, you can do a long, full-body sensate focus exercise in which you begin at the crown chakra and caress each chakra for fifteen minutes or so. The best way to caress each chakra is to move in a slow circular motion. You will channel sexual energy to your partner's genitals if you caress the crown of the head, the forehead, the throat, the heart, the navel, and the pelvis. Then have your partner turn over and lie on his or her stomach so you can caress the base of the spine. After you are done, switch roles. Then you can move into a more sexual activity such as oral sex or intercourse.

♀ Exercise ♂
Tantric Intercourse

According to tantric teaching there is a tremendous store of psychosexual energy that is locked or dormant in the root center at the base of the spine. Tantrics describe it as a coiled serpent named Kundalini.

When you become sexually aroused, this kundalini energy starts to uncoil and slowly move up your spinal cord, energizing the other centers as it goes. You may experience this as a white light or as heat moving along your spine, or as actual sensations of muscular flexing and movement.

To awaken kundalini energy, make love in a straight back position, that is sitting or standing with your spine straight. Try the position with your partner, then the next time you make love switch positions so your partner can experience this. Make sure you come together in a grounding embrace (see the next exercise) after any tantric intercourse.

Raising kundalini energy can be a profound and beautiful experience. It can also make you disoriented and anxious. If it is something you decide to attempt more than occasionally, find a guide or instructor for this essentially spiritual practice.

Raising kundalini is the opposite of the chakra massage described above, in the sense that you begin by stimulating sexual energy and then visualize and experience that energy flowing into the higher chakras. In the chakra massage exercise you began by stimulating the higher centers and allowed the energy to flow to the base of the spine.

Sexual Ecstasy

As you and your partner may have already discovered, there is a level of sexual experience beyond arousal, and even beyond mutuality or intimacy. This is ecstasy. Sexual ecstasy is the feeling that you and your partner are so close during a sexual encounter that you temporarily transcend the material, physical plane of existence and enter into a transcendent realm as you have intercourse and orgasm together.

The way to find ecstasy together is to find balance between the male and female parts of yourselves. A couple will experience love together by learning to transmit that love and respect to each other through their genitals. You will accomplish this by your presence with each other and with your loving intentions.

The exercises in this book lay the foundation for the loving mindset necessary to understand and open the door to ecstasy. Spiritual experiences are always unique and highly personal, so I won't attempt to describe a "typical" ecstatic moment. Some people say they experience intense colors or images, some have visions, others hear music, and some feel an overwhelming sense of connection with all creation. You now have all the tools to use your loving connection as a gateway to the spiritual part of yourself and to connect with the soul of your partner.

The following three exercises are ways that lead to the planes of sexual ecstasy.

♀ Exercise ♂
Intercourse Exchanging Breath

Let's have the man active first. After he has done some sensual caresses with his partner, he kneels between his partner's legs and begins intercourse. As he continues to thrust slowly and sensuously, he leans over his partner and breathes into her mouth. As he breathes out, he visualizes the breath flowing into his partner's lungs, through her body and back into him through her vagina and up his spine. His partner, breathing in, visualizes the same thing. This creates a sensational energy circle that you both can feel.

When the woman is active, she caresses her partner and, when he has a partial or full erection, she climbs on top. As she slowly and sensuously begins to thrust, she breathes into his mouth and they both visualize that the loving breath is flowing into his lungs, abdomen, and pelvis, and through his penis back into her and up her spine. With this visualization, your breath becomes a golden light that fills you both until you feel it radiating outwards.

This can be a very intense exercise, especially if both partners have an orgasm. So, take time to come down from it, at your own pace, and keep close to each other. You might want to end by lying in a close, grounding embrace (see the end of this section) until both of you are ready to release your touch.

♀ Exercise ♂
Eye Gaze Intercourse

In this exercise, you and your partner use your gaze to connect as intimately as you do with your bodies.

Begin by caressing each other as you keep your eyes open and locked onto each other. Gaze deeply into your partner's eyes at the moment of penetration, and as you start to move, stroking up and down, in and out. As your sexual energies build, draw them up and exchange them with your eyes. Keep your movements sensuous and force your partner to look back at you with the power of the sexual energy you create. See if you can stay this focused leading up to and during climax. After you come down from orgasm, lie together in a grounding embrace.

♀ Exercise ♂
Palm Energy and Breath Sharing

This exercise is an enhanced version of an exercise introduced in Chapter 2, and you and your partner may have discovered it spontaneously already. The exercise may sound innocuous, but the combination of palm energy and breath sharing creates an energy exchange that takes you to an altered state of consciousness.

The Exercise Sit cross-legged, facing each other. Gaze lovingly into each other's eyes and do not waver. Raise your hands and place your palms against each other and keep them there for ten seconds. Feel the heat running between you. Now slowly move your hands apart so that they no longer touch but are just close enough so that you can feel a current of energy flow between you.

Concentrating on that flow, lean together as if you were going to kiss. Keep your faces close enough together so that you feel your partner's breath. When one of you breathes in, the other should breathe out. Visualize that breath flowing in a circle: from your mouth to your lungs to your stomach to your pelvis and flowing back into your partner and up through his or her pelvis, stomach, chest, throat and mouth. Now try to reverse this energy circle.

♀ Exercise ♂
Wheel of Love

This is a complicated but very satisfying and energizing exercise that combines all of the elements you have learned in this book—bonding, sensate focus, verbal communication, peaking, plateauing, multiple orgasm, and tantra. Begin with back caresses, front caresses, genital caresses, and oral sex. This exercise can begin with either partner on top. Let's say the man is on top first.

The woman should lie on her back and the man should kneel between her legs. He can caress her vagina with his penis, and enter her when he is ready. At this point, they begin intercourse and they both begin to peak. They should keep their eyes locked on each other. When they reach a strong level of arousal, they should make a small adjustment in their position so that they are now lying on their sides. At the next peak, they should adjust positions again so that the woman is now on top. When they peak and adjust positions again, they will be on their sides again, and after the final position change they will be in the position they started in, with the man kneeling between the woman's legs. It is essential that the couple remains sexually connected for each position change.

Can you visualize what is happening here? As they continue to peak and get more aroused, they are also changing positions so that they are revolving in a wheel. What you have to visualize is that both the man and the woman are becoming more and more aroused, so that by the time they are back to the original position, they are both on the edge of orgasm.

There are a number of variations on this exercise. The version I described above is the simplest way of doing the exercise. You could begin with the woman on top. Or you could begin with the man kneeling, but adjust your legs so that halfway through the exercise you end up in a rear entry position rather than with the woman on top. Rather than changing positions at each peak, you could change positions every few strokes so that you feel as if you are constantly revolving. This is when you really get the sense that you are in "the wheel". The exercise will be more arousing and more satisfying the more you are able to make your movements fluid and seamless. When you have practiced this exercise a number of times, you will find that you can plateau in each position or even orgasm in each position.

♀ Exercise ♂
Grounding Embrace

After any tantric exercise or ecstatic sex, it is very important to center yourselves, or "get grounded." After experiencing altered states of consciousness during intercourse, you won't feel like having a cigarette, taking a shower, or rolling over and going to sleep. You may feel wide-awake and vulnerable, and you probably will not feel like talking.

A good way to come down is through a grounding embrace. It is similar to the Eye Gaze bonding exercise in Chapter 2: lie quietly together face to face, hugging and holding each other, and simply gaze into each other's eyes. Let your breathing slow down naturally, let your energy naturally dissipate, and feel your hearts beat.

This is a lovely finish to the whole ecstatic experience. You will often find that as your breathing and heart rates slow, they fall into sync with each other.

Conclusion

When it comes to making love, there are many aspects that are intangible. We have talked a lot in this book about the "sex" aspects of sexual loving: the type of touch that conveys love, sensuality and desire, how to develop your sexual fitness, how to increase your arousal and sexual potential through peaking and plateauing, how to have multiple orgasms, and more. But there is more to your loving sexual relationship than can be contained by techniques and exercises. I hope you have been able to experience some of that unique, soulful passion—and that the two of you will pursue it!

In closing, I would like to say a few words about the "love" aspects of sexual loving. Very few of us can say what love is, but by the time we're 40 years old or more, we have become comfortable saying that we know what love isn't, and that we know love when we feel it. Part of this may be as a result of our growing experiences in romantic love. Part of it may be wisdom gained from observing the world around us. Part of it may be from raising a family and knowing what it is like to pass on life to our children. I suspect it is because of all of these and a little bit more: as we mature, perhaps it is possible that our thinking brain gives way to our feeling heart as the directing principle or center of our lives.

When you embarked on this journey of sexual loving, you agreed to concentrate on and interact with each other in the moment, not the past or the future. The mutuality and commitment that you showed in doing this was an act of the heart, an act of love. May your love add its light to the good love already out there in the world, making it much, much better than ever.

References

Ainsworth, M.; Blehar, M.; Waters, E.; & Wall, S. *Patterns of Attachment: A Psychological Study of the Strange Situation*. Hillsdale, NJ: Erlbaum, 1978.

Anand, M. *The Art of Sexual Ecstasy*. Los Angeles: Jeremy P. Tarcher, 1989.

Anand, M. *The Art of Sexual Magic*. New York: G. P. Putnam's Sons, 1995.

Bershcheid, E., & Walter, E. "A Little Bit about Love." In *Foundations of Interpersonal Attraction (T. L. Huston)*. New York: Academic Press, 1974.

Buss, D. *The Evolution of Desire: Strategies of Human Mating*. New York: Basic Books, 1994.

Davis, E. *Women, Sex and Desire: Exploring Your Sexuality at Every Stage of Your Life*. Alameda, CA: Hunter House, Inc., 1995.

Hazen, C.; Shaver, P. "Romantic Love Conceptualized as an Attachment Process." In *Journal of Personality and Social Psychology*: 52, 511–524 (1987).

Hendrick, C., Hendrick, S. "A Theory And Method of Love." In *Journal of Personality and Social Psychology*. 56, 392–402 (1986).

Keesling, B. *Sexual Pleasure*. Alameda, CA: Hunter House, 1993.

Keesling, B. *How to Make Love All Night*. New York: HarperCollins, 1994.

Keesling, B. *Talk Sexy to the One You Love*. New York: HarperCollins, 1996.

Keesling, B. *Super Sexual Orgasm*. New York: HarperCollins, 1997.

Lee, J. *The Colors of Love: An Exploration of the Ways of Loving*. Don Mills, Ontario: New Press, 1973.

Montague, A. *Touching: The Human Significance of the Skin. (3rd Ed.)* New York: Harper & Row, 1986.

Ramsdale, D.; Ramsdale, E. *Sexual Energy Ecstasy: A Practical Guide to Lovemaking Secrets of the East and West*. Playa del Rey, CA: Peak Skill Publishing, 1991.

Rubin, Z. *Liking and Loving: An Invitation to Social Psychology*. New York: Holt, Rinehart & Winston, 1973.

Schachter, S. *The Psychology of Affiliation*. Stanford, CA: Stanford University Press, 1959.

Schachter, S.; Singer, J. "Cognitive, Social and Physiological Determinants of Emotional State." In *Psychological Review* (1962): 69, 379–399.

Sternberg, R. "A Triangular Theory of Love." In *Psychological Review* (1986): 93, 119–135.

Index